CLINICAL USE OF LOCAL ANESTHETICS

Edited by **Asadolah Saadatniaki**

Clinical Use of Local Anesthetics
Edited by Asadolah Saadatniaki

Published by InTech
Janeza Trdine 9, 51000 Rijeka, Croatia

Publishing Process Manager Maja Jukic

Technical Editor Teodora Smiljanic

Cover Designer InTech Design Team

Additional hard copies can be obtained from orders@intechopen.com

Clinical Use of Local Anesthetics, Edited by Asadolah Saadatniaki
p. cm.
ISBN 978-953-51-0430-8

For EU product safety concerns:
IN TECH d.o.o., Prolaz Marije Krucifikse Kozulić 3, 51000 Rijeka, Croatia,
info@intechopen.com or visit our website at intechopen.com.

Meet the editor

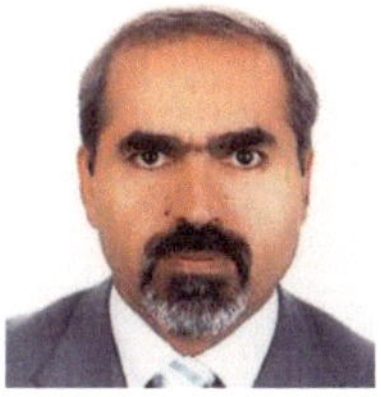

Dr. Asadollah Saadatniaki was born in 1957 in Iran. He graduated as a general physician in 1983 at the Tabriz Medical University, and in 1988 he earned his degree as an anesthesiologist from the Shahid Beheshti Medical University, Tehran, Iran. He has been working in the field of acute pain management since 1990 and from 1999 has actively focused on chronic pain management. From 2001 to 2005 he was a member of the Iranian Anesthesiologist Board Examination. Since 2007, he has been the Director of Pain education program in Shahid Beheshti University of Medical Sciences. Dr. Saadatniaki's scientific activities are in the field of anesthesiology and acute and chronic pain management. The results of his research were presented in different local and international congresses and published in various domestic and international medical journals from 1989 till 2011.

Contents

Preface

From the time of cocaine as the first local anesthetic till now, many local anesthetics have been introduced to clinical practice. Pharmacologic properties of local anesthetics, such as pharmacokinetic and pharmacodynamic properties, have progressed toward the shorter onset, longer duration, higher potency and lower side effects in newer local anesthetics.

Alongside the pharmacologic advancement in newer drugs, clinicians are innovatively utilizing local anesthetics in different fields and in unique states for various surgeries.

This book is an effort to gather the application of local anesthetics in various surgical procedures such as dentistry, plastic surgery, liposuction, hair transplantation, herniorrhaphy and urologic and orthopedic surgeries that are based on the experience of the authors. These local anesthetics have been applied as topical gel, ointment, spray, and so forth.

By considering the content of this book, we think that other procedures which are performed by the use of local anesthetics, such as minimally invasive spinal surgeries, arthroscopy, endovascular procedures and veterinary operations, have the indication for further studies in future clinical trial surveys.

Asadollah Saadatniaki, M.D
Associate Professor of Anesthesiology
Director of Pain Education Program in Shahid Beheshti
University of Medical Sciences, Tehran,
Iran

Acknowledgement

I greatly appreciate the contribution of my colleague Dr. Alireza Mirkheshti, for his assistance in reviewing the chapter proposals.

1

A New and Enhanced Version of Local Anesthetics in Dentistry

Tülin Satılmış, Onur Gönül,
Hasan Garip and Kamil Göker
Faculty of Dentistry, Department of Oral and Maxillofacial Surgery
Marmara University, Istanbul
Turkey

1. Introduction

Pain is an unpleasant sensory and emotional experience associated with actual or potential tissue damage or described in terms of such damage. Due to the fear of pain associated with dental injections, some people avoid, cancel, or fail to appear for dental appointments. Pain and anxiety control are among the most important aspects in local anesthetic administration in dental practice. Administration of local anesthetic produces pain and anxiety that may cause subsequent unfavorable behavior (1). As reliable management of pain is an important factor in reducing fear and anxiety in dental treatment, clinicians must have a thorough knowledge of local anesthetic solutions and techniques. When an agent and a technique are chosen, it is important for the clinician to understand the onset, depth, and duration of anesthesia in relation to the operative procedure to be performed (2). This chapter introduces new local anesthetic formulations, techniques, and postinjection complications in dentistry.

2. Pharmacologic properties of local anesthesia

The main working principle of local anesthetics is to inhibit the ion flow on nerve cell membranes to stabilize membrane potential and block stimulus conduction. Local anesthetics can be defined as compounds capable of reversibly suspending the ability of the nerve tissue to conduct stimuli (3).

Local anesthetics consist of a lipophilic aromatic part, which is responsible for the affinity of the compound to the nerve cells, joined by a connecting chain to a hydrophilic part that is responsible for solubility in water and diffusion among tissues. Decomposition of the compound is affected by the nature of the connecting chain, leading to changes in properties such as duration of action or toxicity. Local anesthetics can be divided into two groups according to the nature of the chemical bonding: esters (*e.g.*, procaine) and amides (*e.g.*, lidocaine) (3–4).

The therapeutic value of such compounds is determined by the typical pharmacological properties of local anesthetics. The compound with the longest history of clinical use, procaine, is used as the basis for comparisons of novel agents. The minimum concentration at which the anesthetic can block stimulus conduction (potency), the therapeutic value of the compound in terms of the correlation between efficacy and tolerability (toxicity), ability of the anesthetic compound to reach tissues at some distance from the site of administration (diffusibility), duration of anesthesia (duration of action), and metabolism of the anesthetic compounds are commonly compared as general pharmacological properties of local anesthetics (3–6).

Vasoconstrictors are added to local anesthetic solutions to inhibit absorption and thus prolong the duration of action and reduce the toxicity of anesthetics as well as to achieve a suitable blood-free area for surgery. Therefore, it is necessary to take into consideration that reactive vasodilatation may occur after surgery with usage of local anesthetics with added vasoconstrictors (7–8).

Adrenaline is the most commonly used vasoconstrictor worldwide. Local anesthetic solutions generally contain adrenaline at a concentration of 1 part per 100000 or 1 part per 200000, resulting in a final content of 0.01–0.005 mg in 1 mL of anesthetic solution. Thus, anesthetic solutions contain adrenaline at very low concentrations compared to the levels required for general physiological effects in healthy individuals (0.3–0.5 mg by subcutaneous administration). There is a great deal of controversy regarding contraindications for the use of adrenaline-containing anesthetics. The mode of administration and quantity added must also be taken into consideration. The American Dental Association and American Heart Association recommend an upper limit of 0.2 mg of adrenaline to be administered in dental operations. On the other hand, the low potency of anesthetic solutions without adrenaline may lead to pain and elevated levels of stress during the operation, resulting in enhanced release of catecholamine (8).

Noradrenaline is another vasoconstrictor used in anesthetic solutions, which has a much weaker local vasoconstrictor effect than adrenaline. Noradrenaline is therefore applied at higher concentrations in anesthetic solutions. The most important advantage of noradrenaline is that it has no direct effect on the cardiovascular system (6–8).

3. Clinical properties of local anesthetics

This section discusses the characteristic clinical properties of the most commonly used local anesthetics.

Procaine: Procaine was synthesized by Einhorn in 1905 and is important in the history of the development of local anesthetics, as it was the first compound to be used in humans. Although it has been superceded in dental practice by more effective modern drugs, the clinical properties of such drugs are still compared with those of procaine as a baseline. Procaine is weaker than modern products currently in use in clinical practice. It is highly soluble in water, and its hydrochloride salt is used as a local anesthetic. It has a low toxicity level and a relatively short duration of action (3,7).

Lidocaine: Lidocaine is currently the most widely used local anesthetic in clinical practice throughout the world. First synthesized by Löfgren and Lundquist in 1943, its potency is fourfold greater than that of procaine, and its toxicity is double that of procaine. The duration of action of lidocaine is double that of procaine, and it shows good diffusibility (4).

Articaine: This preparation, introduced to medical practice by Muschavek and Rippel in 1974, has similar potency, toxicity, and duration of action to lidocaine. Articaine is used almost exclusively in dental practice (7).

Bupivacaine: The toxicity of bupivacaine is ten times that of procaine and has a longer duration of action than lidocaine (7).

Mepivacaine: The potency and toxicity of mepivacaine are similar to those of lidocaine. This agent has a mild vasoconstrictor effect, which leads to a prolonged duration of action (5,6).

Prilocaine: Prilocaine is used in dentistry as a 4% solution containing a vasoconstrictor. This agent has potency equivalent to that of procaine and a toxicity level slightly lower than that of lidocaine and 1.5 times that of procaine (7).

4. Methodology of local anesthesia

Local anesthesia can be classified into two groups according to the manner in which the clinician wants to reach the nerve elements to be anesthetized. The term terminal anesthesia, also called infiltration anesthesia, is used to explain the mode of anesthesia in which the nerve elements are reached at their organ endings, such as the tooth and the periodontal membrane. Practically, there are a number of variants, *i.e.*, topical anesthesia, submucosal infiltration, intramucosal infiltration, and block anesthesia. The term block anesthesia is used to explain blocking of peripheral nerve conduction along the nerve's course. The anesthetic solution is administered at a site some distance from where the clinician wishes to apply the anesthesia (6,7,8,12).

4.1 Anesthesia of upper teeth

In accordance with the maxillary bone structure, anesthesia of the upper teeth is generally performed terminally. The maxilla is covered by a thin cortical layer, and the internal structure of the bone is sponge-like, which facilitates diffusion of local anesthetic solution. The alternative possibility is the nerve-block method, which can be performed in some cases after careful consideration of the advantages and associated risks (7).

4.2 Anesthesia of lower teeth

In contrast to the maxilla, the anatomic structural properties of the mandible force the practitioner to utilize nerve-block anesthesia methods instead of terminal anesthesia. The cortical bone layer that surrounds the mandible is thicker than the maxilla, and the nerve fibers lie in deeper bone structures, leading to poor performance of terminal anesthesia because of the lack of diffusion of the anesthetic solution into deeper parts of the mandible. Therefore, it is essential to be familiar with the anatomical structures and supply areas of the nerves to be affected when performing local anesthesia in the mandible. There is still disagreement regarding whether terminal or nerve block anesthesia is the most appropriate method for the lower incisors (9–11).

4.3 Complications of local anesthesia

Although local anesthesia is commonly defined as a safe and noninvasive procedure, some complications have been reported that can be classified into two groups: general and local (7).

General complications are related to the nature and composition of the local anesthetic solution. The most important general complications are toxic and allergic in nature, both of which are capable of causing death in severe cases. Toxic reactions are rarely seen in dentistry, as the quantities of anesthetic agents applied in dentistry and oral surgery are generally within safe limits. If overdosing occurs, central nervous system effects predominate, and spasms, loss of consciousness, and respiratory depression may occur. It is important not to confuse the overdose reactions with those caused by vasoconstrictors. Allergic reactions are the other most important general complications of local anesthesia. Although allergic reactions caused by local anesthetic solutions with amide linkages are extremely rare, clinicians should always be aware of the symptoms of allergic reactions, especially in patients with a history of polysensitivity to other compounds (11–14).

The most common local complications of local anesthesia in dentistry and oral surgery practice are hematoma, nerve damage, trismus, facial paralysis, and tongue and lip injuries. These local complications may be due to the method of anesthesia used, injury to adjacent anatomical structures, or administration of local anesthetic to an inappropriate site (11–14).

4.4 Volume of local anesthesia

Local anesthesia is not always effective in dentistry. The success of inferior alveolar nerve block ranges from 53% to 100%. A higher degree of success would be expected with infiltration anesthesia. Nevertheless, infiltration injection is not always 100% successful. This can be explained by differences in the smoothness, density, porosity, and thickness of the bone surrounding the maxillary teeth, as well as by individual variations in response to the drug administered. When only the anterior maxilla teeth are considered for the anesthetic, the local anesthetic volume ranges from 0.5 to 1.8 mL (2). Brunetto *et al.* reported that 1.2 mL of 2% lidocaine + 1:100000 epinephrine induced faster onset of pulpal anesthesia, a higher success rate, and a longer duration of soft tissue/pulpal anesthesia of the maxilla (2). Cowan suggested that doses of less than 0.75 mL of 2% lidocaine + 1:80000 epinephrine were adequate for two adjacent teeth after maxillary infiltration. Noncontinuous anesthesia has been reported by other groups after inferior alveolar nerve block. This may be the result of the equilibrium between ionized and nonionized forms of the anesthetic, which results in periods of inadequate pulpal anesthesia (15).

5. Formulation

Inferior alveolar nerve (IAN) block is the most frequently used method for achieving local anesthesia for mandibular procedures. However, IAN block does not always result in successful pulpal anesthesia. Local anesthetics are chemical compounds that cause reversible blockade of nerve impulses. They are weak bases with pKa values between 7.5 and 9.0, and their physicochemical properties largely determine their clinical anesthetic characteristics. Galindo *et al.* used pH-adjusted local anesthetic solutions (pH 7.4) in peripheral nerve block and regional anesthesia and reported better quality of anesthesia (16). Davies reviewed the relevant literature and concluded that buffering local anesthetics with sodium bicarbonate significantly reduced injection pain (17).

Whitcomb *et al.* reported that buffering 2% lidocaine + 1:100000 epinephrine with 0.17 mEq/mL sodium bicarbonate did not significantly increase the success of anesthesia, provide faster onset, or result in less pain at injection compared with unbuffered 2% lidocaine + 1:100000 epinephrine for inferior alveolar nerve block. They considered raising the pH of the anesthetic formulation to 7.9, which is the acid dissociation constant (pKa) of lidocaine, thereby producing equal amounts of the cation and the base form. However, a pilot study of various formulations demonstrated irritating effects (cellulitis and tissue injury). They found that a concentration of 0.17 mEq/mL of sodium bicarbonate raised the pH of the lidocaine formulation to 7.5 without causing an irritating effect. They used a total volume of 3.6 mL of the lidocaine/sodium bicarbonate formulation to allow more sodium bicarbonate to be used by volume than a volume of 1.8 mL would have allowed. Each subject received 72 mg of lidocaine by administration of unbuffered lidocaine, while use of buffered lidocaine resulted in administration of only 60 mg of lidocaine. Therefore, subjects in the buffered group received 17% less lidocaine. Although less lidocaine was administered to patients receiving the buffered formulation, the same success rate of anesthesia was achieved as with the unbuffered lidocaine formulation (18).

Maxillary and mandibular infiltration anesthesia is a common method of anesthetizing maxillary and mandibular teeth. Katz *et al.* reported that success of anesthesia and onset of pulpal anesthesia were not significantly different among 2% lidocaine + 1:100000 epinephrine, 4% prilocaine + 1:200000 epinephrine, and 4% prilocaine for the maxillary lateral incisor and first molar. For both the lateral incisor and first molar, 4% prilocaine + 1: 200000 epinephrine and 2% lidocaine + 1: 100000 epinephrine showed equivalent pulpal anesthesia. However, neither agent provided 1 hour of pulpal anesthesia. For both the lateral incisor and first molar, 4% prilocaine provided a significantly shorter duration of pulpal anesthesia compared with 2% lidocaine + 1: 100000 epinephrine and 4% prilocaine + 1:200000 epinephrine. Katz *et al.* suggested that the infiltration injection of 1.8 mL of 2% lidocaine + 1: 100000 epinephrine may not always be 100% successful because of individual variations in response to the drug administered, operator differences, and variations in anatomy and tooth position. The success rate of the infiltration of 4% prilocaine + 1: 200000 epinephrine was 90% in the lateral incisor and 93% in the first molar. The success of the infiltration of 4% prilocaine was 83% in the lateral incisor and 80% in the first molar and provided a shorter duration of pulpal anesthesia (19).

The mandible is comprised of dense, thick cortical bone, and the efficacy of infiltration anesthesia for mandibular molars in dental procedures has therefore traditionally been considered inadequate. Abdulwahab *et al.* evaluated the efficacy of six local anesthetic formulations (2% lidocaine + 1:100000 epinephrine (L100), 4% articaine + 1:200000 epinephrine (A200), 4% articaine + 1:100000 epinephrine (A100), 4% prilocaine + 1:200000 epinephrine (P200), 3% mepivacaine without vasoconstrictor (Mw/o), and 0.5% bupivacaine + 1:200000 epinephrine (B200) used for posterior mandibular buccal infiltration anesthesia. They showed that the maximum mean increases from baseline EPT measurements for the six formulations were 43.5% for L100, 44.8% for B200, 51.2% for P200, 66.9% for A200, 68.3% for Mw/o, and 77.3% for A100 (A100 *vs.* L100, $P = 0.029$). They reported that the mean VAS pain ratings for injection pain were 32.2 for B200, 27.6 for L100, 26.2 for A100, 24.1 for A200, 22.9 for Mw/o, and 21.0 for P200 (20).

Inferior alveolar nerve block (IANB) is the most frequently used injection technique for achieving local anesthesia for mandibular restorative and surgical procedures. In asymptomatic patients, inferior alveolar nerve block fails 17–19% of the time in the first molar. Therefore, it would be advantageous to improve the success rate of the IANB technique. Additionally, slow onset of anesthesia occurs 12–19% of the time in the first molar with IANB and the use of articaine or lidocaine solutions. If supplemental buccal infiltration can reduce the failure rate and increase the speed of onset of pulpal anesthesia after IANB, the technique may be clinically useful. Haase *et al.* compared the anesthetic efficacy of articaine *vs.* lidocaine as supplemental buccal infiltration of the mandibular first molar after inferior alveolar nerve block. They found that with use of the 4% articaine + 1:100000 epinephrine formulation, successful pulpal anesthesia was achieved for the first molar in 88% of cases. With the 2% lidocaine + 1:100000 epinephrine formulation, successful pulpal anesthesia occurred in 71% of cases (21). Robertson and colleagues compared the degree of pulpal anesthesia achieved with mandibular first molar buccal infiltration of 4% articaine + 1:100000 epinephrine and 2% lidocaine + 1:100000 epinephrine. Using the lidocaine formulation, they achieved a success rate of 57% for the first molar. Using the articaine formulation, they achieved successful pulpal anesthesia in 87% of cases. The differences in rates achieved with 2% lidocaine and 4% articaine formulations were significant ($P < 0.05$). Therefore, 4% articaine + 1:100000 epinephrine is superior to 2% lidocaine + 1:100000 epinephrine in mandibular buccal infiltration of the first molar. However, Robertson and colleagues found that pulpal anesthesia with both the 4% articaine and 2% lidocaine formulations declined slowly over 60 minutes (22). Foster *et al.* investigated the anesthetic efficacy of buccal and lingual infiltrations of lidocaine following inferior alveolar nerve block in mandibular posterior teeth. They found that adding buccal or lingual infiltration of 1.8 mL of 2% lidocaine + 1:100000 epinephrine to IANB did not significantly increase the success of anesthesia in mandibular posterior teeth (23).

Pabst *et al.* investigated the efficacy of repeated buccal infiltration of articaine in prolonging the duration of pulpal anesthesia in the mandibular first molar. The degree of pulpal anesthesia obtained with two sets of mandibular first molar buccal infiltrations given in two separate doses was examined in 86 adult subjects: an initial infiltration of a cartridge of 4% articaine + 1:100000 epinephrine plus a second infiltration of the same anesthetic and dose 25 minutes after the initial infiltration *vs.* an initial infiltration of a cartridge of 4% articaine + 1:100000 epinephrine plus mock repeat infiltration given 25 minutes following the initial infiltration. The authors used an electric pulp tester to test the first molar for anesthesia in 3-minute cycles for 112 minutes after the injections. The repeated infiltration significantly improved pulpal anesthesia from 28 minutes to 109 minutes in the mandibular first molar. Repeated infiltration of a cartridge of 4% articaine + 1:100000 epinephrine given 25 minutes after the initial infiltration of the same type and dose of anesthetic significantly improved the duration of pulpal anesthesia in the mandibular first molar compared with initial buccal infiltration alone (24).

Increasing attention has been focused on the clinical application of α-2 adrenoceptor agonists for anesthetic management. Furthermore, various methods of administration, such as epidural, intrathecal, and peripheral injections, have been examined alone or in combination with another drug to prolong and intensify the anesthesia. The α-2 adrenoceptor agonist, clonidine, combined with a local anesthetic, has been found to extend the duration of peripheral nerve block. The action of clonidine was suggested to be due to local vasoconstriction and/or direct inhibition of impulse conduction in peripheral nerves. However, the mechanism of action has not been fully elucidated. Clonidine is not particularly specific to α-2 adrenoceptors and also acts *via* α-1 adrenoceptors at comparatively high concentrations. Clonidine has the ability to induce vasoconstriction, and it is therefore unclear whether it acts *via* α-2 adrenoceptors. On the other hand, another α-2 adrenoceptor agonist, dexmedetomidine, acts more specifically against α-2 adrenoceptors and has more than eight times greater affinity for α-2 adrenoceptors of clonidine(25). It has sedative, analgesic, and sympatholytic effects that blunt many of the cardiovascular responses(hypertension, tachycardia) seen during the perioperative period (26). Dexmedetomidine has also been reported to enhance central and peripheral neural blockaded by local anesthetics; however, the peripheral effects have not been fully clarified. Yoshitomi *et al.* reported that dexmedetomidine and other α-2 adrenoceptor agonists (oxymetazoline hydrochloride, yohimbine hydrochloride, prazosin hydrochloride) enhanced the local anesthetic action of lidocaine in the periphery (25).

Ketamine is a well-known general anesthetic and short-acting intraoperative analgesic. Ketamine has multiple effects throughout the central nervous system, including blocking polysynaptic reflexes in the spinal cord and inhibiting excitatory neurotransmitter effects in selected areas of the brain. It dissociates the thalamus (which relays sensory impulses from the reticular activating system to the cerebral cortex) from the limbic cortex (which is involved with the awareness of sedation). While some brain neurons are inhibited, others are tonically excited. Clinically, this state of dissociative anesthesia causes the patient to appear conscious (eg, eye opening, swallowing, muscle contracture) but unable to process or respond to sensory input (26).This agent is a nonselective antagonist of supraspinal *N*-methyl-D-aspartate (NMDA) receptors, which are activated by the excitatory neurotransmitter glutamate. Inhibition of NMDA receptors decreases neuronal signaling and is likely responsible for some of the analgesic effects of ketamine. Satilmis *et al.* demonstrated that the combination of a local anesthetic and subanesthetic doses of ketamine during surgical extraction of third molars can produce good local anesthesia while affording a comfortable procedure for both surgeon and patient, providing good postoperative analgesia with reduced swelling and significantly less trismus than local anesthesia alone (27).

Failure to achieve anesthesia can be a significant problem in dental practice. Studies have shown that more than 50% of adults in the USA miss dentistry services because of a fear of pain. Controlling patients' anxiety and distress, good treatment of root canals, effective use of local anesthetics, and drug therapy cover the main factors in the management of dental pain. Amitriptyline is one of the most common tricyclic antidepressants (TCAs) and binds to pain sensory nerve fibers close to the sodium channels; hence, it may interact to some degree with receptors of local anesthetics. Although TCAs have been successfully used in the treatment of some types of neuropathic pain and they have been shown to have efficacy in blocking Na channels in the nervous system, they have not been used systemically for the completion of anesthesia in dental pain because of the potential risks of adverse drug reactions. However, topical use of a lipid-soluble TCA, *e.g.*, amitriptyline, administered directly into the pulp cavity of a painful tooth in addition to routine local anesthetic injection may synergistically complete analgesia through coinhibition of Na channels on pain sensory fibers. Moghadamnia *et al.* reported that inter-pulp-space administration of 2% amitriptyline gel for completing analgesia in irreversible pulpitis pain was effective and useful as a conjunctive therapy to injection of local anesthetics (28).

6. References

[1] Shahidi Bonjar AH. Syringe micro vibrator (SMV) a new device being introduced in dentistry to alleviate pain and anxiety of intraoral injections, and a comparative study with a similar device. Ann Surg Innov Res. 2011;5:1.

[2] Brunetto PC, Ranali J, Ambrosano GM, *et al.* Anesthetic efficacy of 3 volumes of lidocaine with epinephrine in maxillary infiltration anesthesia. Anesth Prog. 2008; 55(2):29–34.

[3] Milam SB, Giovannitti JA Jr. Local anesthetics in dental practice. Dent Clin North Am. 1984;28(3):493–508.

[4] Sisk AL. Vasoconstrictors in local anesthesia for dentistry. Anesth Prog. 1992;39(6):187–93.

[5] MacKenzie TA, Young ER. Local anesthetic update. Anesth Prog. 1993;40(2):29–34.

[6] Yagiela JA. Recent developments in local anesthesia and oral sedation. Compend Contin Educ Dent. 2004;25(9):697–706; quiz 708.

[7] Szabo G. In: Oral & Maxillofacial Surgery. Semmelweis Publishing House. Budapest 2001. p. 20–34

[8] Moore PA, Hersh EV. Local anesthetics: pharmacology and toxicity. Dent Clin North Am. 2010;54(4):587–99.

[9] Berlin J, Nusstein J, Reader A, Beck M, Weaver J. Efficacy of articaine and lidocaine in a primary intraligamentary injection administered with a computer-controlled local anesthetic delivery system. Oral Surg Oral Med Oral Pathol Oral Radiol Endod. 2005;99(3):361–6.

[10] Hawkins JM, Moore PA. Local anesthesia: advances in agents and techniques. Dent Clin North Am. 2002;46(4):719–32, ix.

[11] Kaufman E, Epstein JB, Naveh E, Gorsky M, Gross A, Cohen G. A survey of pain, pressure, and discomfort induced by commonly used oral local anesthesia injections. Anesth Prog. 2005;52(4):122-7.
[12] Finder RL, Moore PA. Adverse drug reactions to local anesthesia. Dent Clin North Am. 2002;46(4):747-57, x.
[13] Speca SJ, Boynes SG, Cuddy MA. Allergic reactions to local anesthetic formulations. Dent Clin North Am. 2010;54(4):655-64.
[14] Malamed SF. Allergy and toxic reactions to local anesthetics. Dent Today. 2003;22(4):114-6, 118-21.
[15] Cowan A. Minimum dosage technique in the clinical comparison of representative modern local anesthetic agents. *J Dent Res.* 1964;43:1228-49.
[16] Galindo A. pH-adjusted local anesthetics: clinical experience. *Reg Anesth.* 1983;8:35-6.
[17] Davies RJ. Buffering the pain of local anesthetics: a systematic review. *Emerg Med (Fremantle)* 2003;15:81-8.
[18] Whitcomb M, Drum M, Nusstein J, Beck M. A prospective, randomized, double-blind study of the anesthetic efficacy of sodium bicarbonate buffered 2% lidocaine with 1:100,000 epinephrine in inferior alveolar nerve blocks. Anesth Prog 2010; 57(2):59-66.
[19] Katz S, Drum M, Nusstein J, Beck M. A prospective, randomized, double-blind comparison of 2% lidocaine with 1:100,000 epinephrine, 4% prilocaine with 1:200,000 epinephrine, and 4% prilocaine for maxillary infiltrations. Anesth Prog 2010;57(2):45-51.
[20] Abdulwahab M, Boynes S, Moore P, *et al.* The efficacy of six local anesthetic formulations used for posterior mandibular buccal infiltration anesthesia. J Am Dent Assoc. 2009;140(8):1018-24.
[21] Haase A, Nusstein J, Beck M, Drum M. Comparing anesthetic efficacy of articaine versus lidocaine as a supplemental buccal infiltration of the mandibular first molar after an inferior alveolar nerve block. J Am Dent Assoc. 2008;139(9):1228-35.
[22] Robertson D, Nusstein J, Reader A, Beck M, McCartney M. The anesthetic efficacy of articaine in buccal infiltration of mandibular posterior teeth. JADA 2007;138(8):1104-1112.Foster W, Drum M, Beck M. Anesthetic efficacy of buccal and lingual infiltrations of lidocaine following an inferior alveolar nerve block in mandibular posterior teeth. Anesth Prog. 2007;54(4):163-9.
[23] Pabst L, Nusstein J, Drum M, Beck M. The efficacy of a repeated buccal infiltration of articaine in prolonging duration of pulpal anesthesia in the mandibular first molar. Anesth Prog. 2009;56(4):128-34.
[24] Yoshitomi T, Kohjitani A, Maeda S. Dexmedetomidine enhances the local anesthetic action of lidocaine via an α-2a adrenoceptor. Anesth Analg 2008;107(1):96-101.
[25] Morgan GE, Mikhail M, Murray M. In: Clinical Anesthesiology. Lange Medical Books/McGraw-Hill Medical Publishing Division. London. 2002. p 217-218.
[26] Satilmis T, Garip H, Arpaci E, *et al.* Assessment of combined local anesthesia and ketamine for pain, swelling, and trismus after surgical extraction of third molars. J Oral Maxillofac Surg. 2009;67:1206-10.

[27] Moghadamnia AA, Partovi M, Mohammadianfar I *et al*. Evaluation of the effect of locally administered amitriptyline gel as adjunct to local anesthetics in irreversible pulpitis pain. Indian J Dent Res. 2009;20(1):3–6.

2

Local Anesthesia for Cosmetic Procedures

Dhepe V. Niteen
Dermatosurgery Taskforce, IADVL, SkinCity, Post Graduate Institute of Dermatology and Lasers, Solapur, Maharashtra India

1. Introduction

In recent years the number of cosmetic procedures is continuously increasing. Cosmetic procedure/surgery is an elective procedure. It is not an emergency. Hence not only final result but the overall comfort and satisfaction of the patient are equally important. Majority of the procedures are carried out under local anesthesia; so thorough knowledge of local anesthetic agents, types, techniques and their side effects becomes very much important for the aesthetic physicians.

1.1 Learning objectives

At the end of reading of this chapter, reader should be able to understand the scope of various types of local anesthesia in his aesthetic practice, able to choose appropriate local anesthesia according to indication, able to do modification in various techniques according to the demand of situation to give pleasant and comfortable experience to patient during the aesthetic procedure while keeping in mind the possible adverse effects of the anesthesia.

1.2 Mechanism of local anesthetic activity

Studies have shown that local anesthetics inhibit depolarization of the nerve by interfering with the influx of Na^+ ions. Although the exact mechanism of local anesthetic action is not known, several theories postulate that anesthetics diffuse across the neural membrane and somehow alter the activity of the Na^+ channel. Local anesthetics are thought to stabilize the membrane at resting potential, increase the threshold for electrical excitation, and reduce the propagation of an excitatory impulse, thereby blocking nerve conduction.[1]

The sensation of pain is carried via small unmyelinated nerve fibers (C fibers). These fibers are more sensitive to the actions of local anesthetics as compared to larger nerve fibers that carry other sensations. Consequently patients may be able to feel sensations such as pressure and vibration, while being insensitive to pain.[2]

1.3 Classification of local anesthetics

Local anesthetics possess a basic chemical structure that gives it amphipathic characteristics. Its structure can be divided into three distinct parts: an aromatic portion (lipophilic), intermediate chain, and amine group (hydrophilic). The intermediate chain connects the aromatic group to the amine group. It is also the basis of local anesthetic classification as either esters or amides (Table 1).

Ester anesthetics are metabolized via the plasma enzyme, pseudocholinesterase. Hydrolysis is rapid and the by-products are excreted in the urine.

Amide anesthetics are metabolized primarily by the liver. They should be used with caution in patients with liver disease.[3]

For detailed discussion on pharmacology of local anesthetic agents, kindly refer to the related chapter in this book.

Group	Generic name	Trade name	Onset of anesthesia	Duration of anesthesia	Available Concentration (%)
Amides					
	Lidocaine	Xylocaine	Rapid	Moderate	0.5, 1.0, 2.0
	Mepivicaine	Carbocaine	Rapid	Moderate	1.0, 2.0
	Bupivicaine	Marcaine	Slow	Long	0.25, 0.5, 0.75
	Etidocaine	Duranest	Rapid	Long	0.5, 1.0
Esters					
	Procaine	Novacaine	Rapid	Short	0.5, 1.0, 2.0
	Tetracaine	Pontocaine	Slow	Long	0.1,0.25

Table 1. Common Local Anesthetics Used in Dermatology[2, 4]

1.4 Combination of Local anesthetics and adrenaline[5, 6]

Many times local anesthetic is administered along with vasoconstrictor like adrenaline with beneficial results. This combination offers following advantages:

1. Decrease anesthetic absorption and systemic toxicity with improved efficacy and smaller amounts required.
2. Prolonged duration of action (almost doubled), especially with lignocaine and procaine
3. Less bleeding at operative site, especially useful on vascular areas with better visualization of operative field.

Adrenaline may potentially induce adverse effects. Therefore its use must be carefully considered in patients with heart disease and those patients concomitantly taking ß-blockers.[7]

	Symptoms	Treatment
	Central nervous system	
Lidocaine	Drowsiness, circumoral	Intravenous diazepam, oxygen
	numbness, tingling of tongue,	
	metallic taste, diplopia,	
	blurred vision, tinnitus,	
	slurred speech, muscle	
	twitching, shivering, seizure,	
	respiratory arrest	
Epinephrine	Nervousness, tremors,	
	headaches	
	Cardiovascular system	
Lidocaine	Progressive myocardial	Cardiopulmonary,
	depression, prolonged	resuscitation, oxygen,
	conduction time,	vasopressors,
	arteriovenous block,	intravenous fluids
	bradycardia vasomotor	
	depression, hypotension,	
	hypoxia, acidosis	
Epinephrine	Tachycardia, palpitations,	Vasodilators (hydralazine,
	chest pain, hypertension	clonidine, sublingual
		nifedipine)
	Allergic	
Lidocaine	Urticaria, angioedema,	Antihistamines, subcutaneous
	anaphylaxis	epinephrine, oxygen, steroids
	Psychogenic	
		Cold compresses on forehead
	Vasovagal response	and neck, Trendelenburg position,
		fan patient, ammonia ampule

Table 2. Adverse Effects of Lidocaine with Epinephrine[8]

2. Types of local anesthesia for cosmetic procedures

2.1 Topical anesthesia[9]

Topical anesthesia is the surface application of a LA to the skin or mucous membrane by means of a spray, spreading of an ointment,). Lidocaine 2% jelly, EMLA cream, or iontophoresis of lidocaine can allow one to perform simple procedures such as shave biopsies, electro-cauterization of epidermal growths or superficial laser surgery. Topical anesthetics can also provide surface anesthesia to permit painless insertion of a needle, especially in children, and on painful areas such as the nose, lips and genitalia.[10]

2.1.1 Mucosal agents

Topical anesthetics agents are useful on mucosal surfaces include cocaine 4%, benzocaine 5-20%,tetracaine 0.5% and lidocaine 2-5% (jelly, ointment), lidocaine 10% aerosol etc.

2.1.2 Cutaneous agents

Creams: for producing an anesthesia on intact skin, creams of lidocaine (30%) or EMLA – eutectic mixture of local anesthetics have to be applied for variable period of time (30min to 2 hours) according to the composition of the EMLA. This EMLA has to be applied under occlusion for its optimum effect. The list of commonly available topical anesthetic is given in Table 3.

Special delivery techniques for topical anesthesia

- Iontophoresis[11]
  The introduction of various ions into the skin through the use of electricity has been increasingly used to provide pain relief in outpatient procedures. It uses an electric current to overcome some of the barriers of the skin and assist the penetration through the movement of ions into the skin via sweat glands, hair follicles and sebaceous glands.
  Iontophoresis can be used to deliver chemicals to both superficial and deeper layers of the skin.
  Advantages are
  1. It avoids pain associated with injections.
  2. It prevents the variation in absorption seen with oral medications
  3. It bypasses first-pass elimination
  4. Drugs with sorter half life can be delivered directly to the tissue

  Disadvantages are
  1. Discomfort and erythema at the site of iontophoresis secondary to pH changes
  2. There is also potential of skin irritation and burn
- Laser assisted delivery of Topical anesthetics:
  A research in 2003 indicates that a single pass of the Er:YAG laser (wave length 2940 nm) enhanced the absorption and penetration of lidocaine by disrupting the stratum corneum.[12]
  Although this technique may not be adequate for invasive procedures, it may minimize pain and discomfort for more superficial cutaneous procedure, such as hypodermic needle insertion. This is a well known fact that reapplication of topical anesthetic after first pass of ablative lasers produce quicker and deeper anesthesia.
  Interest in laser assisted drug delivery was reemerged after advent of fractional lasers. Narrow but deep vertical channels of ablation into skin created by fractional CO2 laser were used to successfully deliver a drug, methyl 5-aminolevulinate (MAL) to a uniform depth into skin.[13] The absoption was uniform and full thickness indicating drug delivery from lateral walls of the tunnel. Currently trials are under progress to use this method to deliver local anesthetic agent to skin.

Anesthetic	Ingredients	Vehicle	Application Dose	Occlusion required	FDA approved	Advantages	Disadvantages	Max Dose/ Area
Betacain-LA	Lidocaine Prilocain Dibucaine	Vaseline ointment	60-90	No	No	Anecdotal reports of rapid onset	more clinical and safty trial needed	$300cm^2$- adults
LMX	4% Lidocaine	Liposomal	60	No	Yes	Liposomal delivery long duration of action	Post application residue	$100cm^2$- children $600cm^2$- 10kg-adult /children
LMX 5	5% Lidocaine	Liposomal	30	No	Yes	Rapid onset of action	more clinical trails needed	$100cm^2$- children $600cm^2$- 10kg-adult /children
EMLA	2.5% Lidocaine 2.5% Prilocain	Oil in water	60	Yes	Yes	Proven efficacy and safety profile	Long application occlusion required	$20g/200cm^2$ adult and children older than 7 and >20 kg
Tretracaine gel	4% Tretracaine Gel	Lecithin gel	60-90	Yes	No	Anecdotal reports of rapid onset	more clinical and safty trial needed	None reported
Amethocaine	4% Tretracaine		40-60	Yes	No	Rapid onset prolonged effect	Ester anesthetic, avoid mucosal surfaces	50mg-adult
Topicaine	4% Lidocaine	Microemulsion	30-60	Yes	Yes	Rapid onset Cost effective	more clinical trial needed	$600cm^2$-adult (children >10kg)
S-Caine	2.5% Lidocaine 2.5% Tretracaine	Oil in water	30-60	No	Phase III clinical trails	Unique delivery system	Contains as Ester anesthetic	To be determined

Table 3. Drugs used for topical anesthesia[14]

- Needle-less Dermajet
  This is a needleless pressure injection syringe for the intradermal infiltration of drugs in a soluble state. This technique achieves almost painless tissue infiltration with a high velocity microspray in single or multiple doses of 0.1 cc. to a depth of 2 to 5 mm. without actual contact with the site of injection. A fine jet emitted under great pressure punctures the tissue without coring, with a minimum amount of trauma, raising instantaneously a well-defined pinpoint wheal. Besides giving local anesthesia this mode of drug delivery is useful in intralesional steroid injection in case of keloid and hypertrophic scar, in mass vaccinations[15] etc.
- Microporation
  Iontophoresis applies a small low voltage (typically 10 V or less) continuous constant current (typically 0.5 mA/cm^2 or less) to push a charged drug into skin or other tissue. In contrast, electroporation applies a high voltage (typically, >100 V) pulse for a very short (μs-ms) duration to permeabilize the skin.[16] Low frequency ultrasound is also used as 'sonoporation'.

2.2 Infiltration anesthesia[9]

This is the most commonly used method of anesthetizing the skin. It consists of injecting the anesthetic agent into the tissue to be cut. The injection may be intradermal, when the anesthesia is almost immediate, or into the subcutaneous tissue, when the anesthesia is usually delayed and has a shorter duration. However, an intradermal injection is more painful. The pain of a LA injection into the skin can be reduced by adding freshly prepared sodium bicarbonate (8.4%) solution to the LA solution in a 1:10 dilution. Local pain can also be reduced by injecting the drug slowly, while pinching the neighboring skin to distract the patient. The infiltration may distort the operative site; this can be minimized by gentle massage after the injection.

2.3 Field blocks[9]

A field or ring block is a variation of infiltration anesthesia. The LA agent is placed around the operative site, anesthetizing the nerve fibers leaving from the area. A ring block is useful when direct needle entry into a lesion such as a cyst is not desirable. The LA has to be placed in both superficial and deep planes. Start injecting from proximal to distal end. This also limits the amount of LA needed to anesthetize the operative site. This is a particular advantage when a large area has to be anesthetized.

2.4 Peripheral nerve blocks

A nerve block involves placing the local anesthetic solution in a specific location at or around the main nerve trunk that will effectively depolarize that nerve and obtund sensation in the area of sensory distribution of that particular nerve. In dermatological surgery, the commonly employed nerve blocks are for the digits and for the central face, because both areas are painful to anesthetize using local infiltration. Peripheral nerve blocks are difficult to perform and complications include laceration of the nerve, intravascular injection of LA and hematoma formation may occur.

Advantages of nerve blocks include the fact that a single accurately placed injection can obtund large areas of sensation without tissue distortion at operative site.

Disadvantages of peripheral nerve blocks include the sensation of numbness in areas other than the operative site and the lack of hemostasis at the operative site from the vasoconstrictor component of the local anesthetic injection.

Since many nerves are accompanied by corresponding veins and arteries, pre-injection aspiration should always be performed to prevent intra vascular injection. Use of local anesthetics with vasoconstrictors will prolong anesthesia.

3. Sensory nerves and respective dermatomes of face and their block

3.1 Fig 1a and 1b Sensory innervations of face and neck area

Trigeminal nerve

Often referred to as "the great sensory nerve of the head and neck", the trigeminal nerve is named for its three major sensory branches. The ophthalmic nerve (VI), maxillary nerve (V2), and mandibular nerve (V3) are literally 'three twins' (trigeminal) carrying sensory information of light touch, temperature, pain, and proprioception from the face and scalp to brainstem. The main branches of the trigeminal nerve supply sensation to the well defined and consistent facial areas.

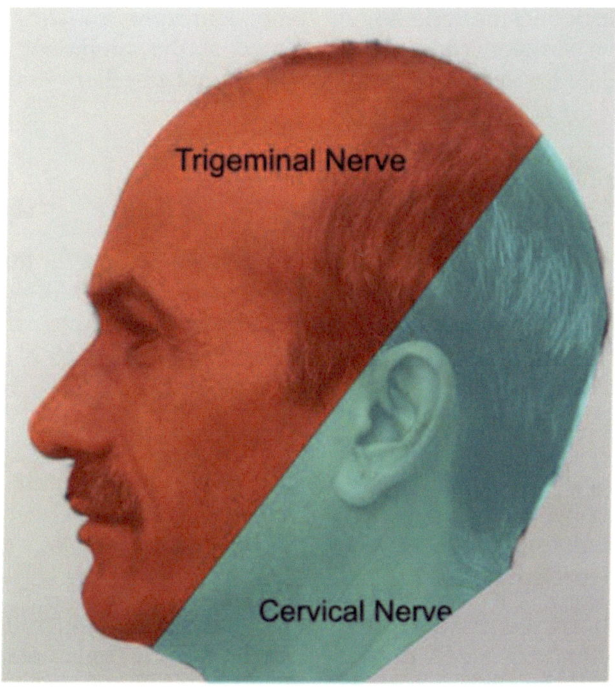

Fig. 1a.

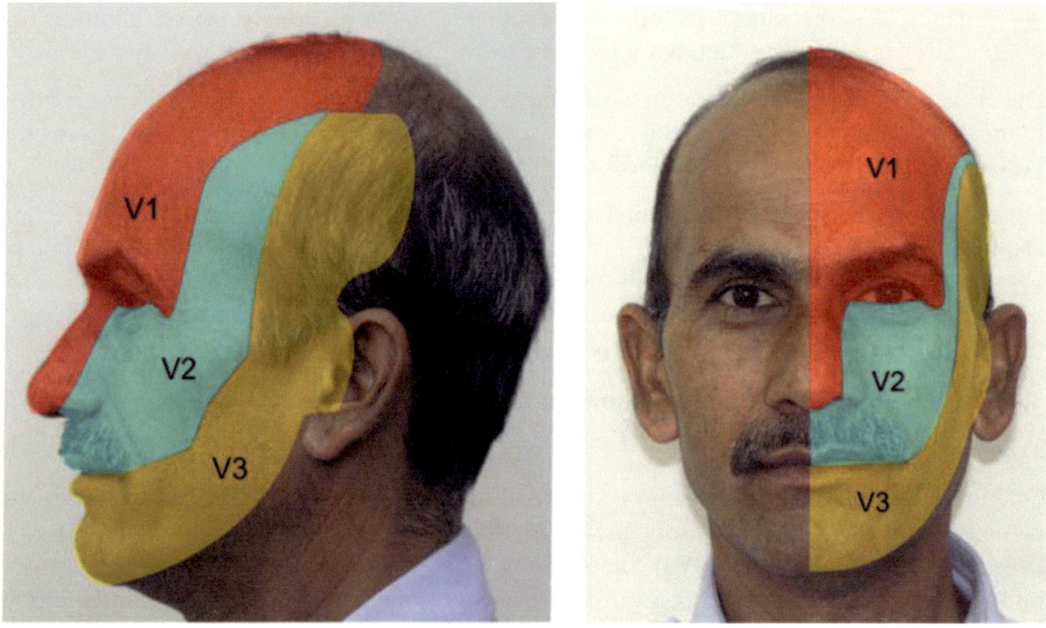

Fig. 1b.

3.2 Anatomic arrangement of facial foramina

Successful nerve block anesthesia is largely dependent upon knowing the position of the nerve foramina. The surgeon can take advantage of the alignment of the major facial foramina as they relate to a vertical line through the mid pupillary line with the eye in the primary position of natural forward gaze.

3.3 Common nerve blocks[17]

1. Supraorbital nerve
   The supraorbital nerve exits through a notch (in some case a foramen) on the superior orbital rim approximately 27 mm lateral to the glabellar midline. This supraorbital notch is readily palpable in most patients. After existing the notch or foramen, the nerve traverses the corrugator supercilii muscles and branches into a medical and lateral portion. The lateral branches supply the lateral forehead and the medial branches supply the scalp.
2. Supratrochlear nerve and Supraorbital
   The supratrochlear nerve exits a foramen approximately 17 mm from the glabellar midline and supplies sensation to the middle portion of the forehead. The infratrochlear nerve exits a foramen below the trochlea and provided sensation to the medial upper eyelid, canthus, medial nasal skin, conjunctiva, and lateral lacrimal apparatus.

When injecting this area it is prudent to always use the nondominant hand to palpate the orbital rim to ensure that the needle tip is exterior to the bony orbital margin. To anesthetize this area, the supratrochlear nerve is measured 17 mm from the glabellar midline and 1-2 mL of local anesthetic is injected. The **supraorbital nerve** is blocked by palpating the notch (and/or measuring 27 mm from the glabellar midline) and injecting 1-2 mL of local anesthetic solution. The infratrochlear nerve is blocked by injecting 1-2 mL of local anesthetic solution at the junction of the orbit and the nasal bones.

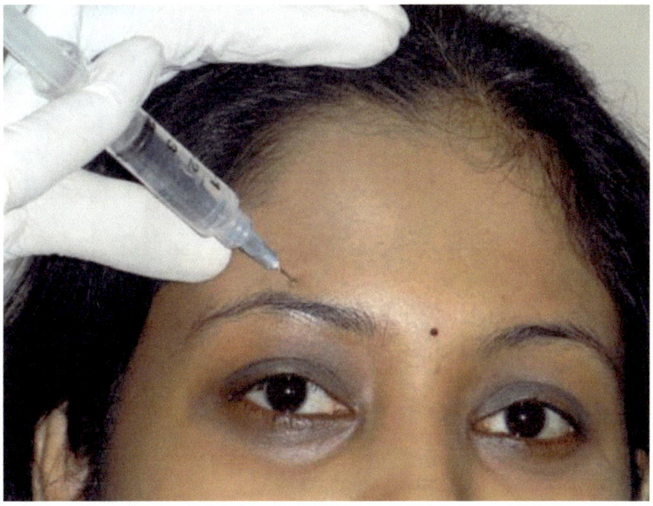

Fig. 2. Supra orbital nerve block

3.4 Infraorbital nerve block

This block is one of the most commonly utilized facial blocks in order to anesthetize the upper lip and upper nasolabial fold for injection of fillers. Obviously, a bilateral block must be performed to achieve anesthesia on both sides of the lip.

The Infraorbital nerve exits the Infraorbital foramen 4-7 mm below the orbital rim in an imaginary line dropped from the midpupillary midline. The anterior superior alveolar nerve branches from the Infraorbital nerve before it exits the foramen, and thus some patients will manifest anesthesia of the anterior teeth and gingival if the branching is closed to the foramen. Areas anesthetized include the lateral nose, anterior cheek, lower eyelid, and upper lip on the injected side. This nerve can be blocked by intraoral or extraoral routes.

To perform an Infraorbital nerve block from an **intraoral** approach, (fig 3) topical anesthesia is placed on the oral mucosa at the vestibular sulcus just under the canine fossa (between the canine and first premolar tooth) and left for several minutes. The lip is then elevated and a ½ inch 30 gauge needle is inserted in the sulcus and directed superiorly towards the Infraorbital foramen. Bending the needle at 45 degree angle upward can facilitate the needle insertion. The needle needs only to approach the vast branching around the foramen to be effective. It is important to use the other hand to palpate the inferior orbital rim to avoid injecting superiorly the orbit. 2-4 mL of 2% lidocaine is injected in this area for the Infraorbital block and the palpating finger can feel the local anesthetic bolus below the Infraorbital rim, confirming the correct are of placement.

The Infraorbital nerve can also be very easily blocked by the **transcutaneous facial approach** and may be the preferred rout in dental phobic patients. (fig 4). A 32 gauge ½ inch needle is used and is placed through the skin and aimed at the foramen in a perpendicular direction. Between 2 and 4 mL of local anesthetic solution is injected at or close to the foramen. Again, the other hand must constantly palpate the inferior orbital rim to prevent inadvertent injection into the orbit. Care must be taken in this approach to avoid superficial vessels that may cause noticeable bruising.

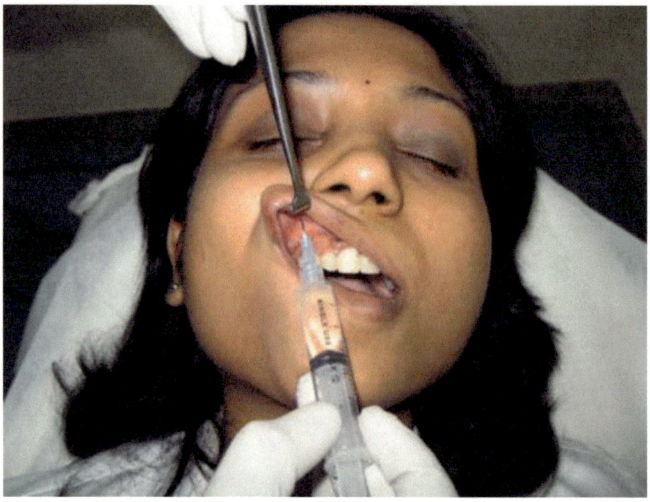

Fig. 3.

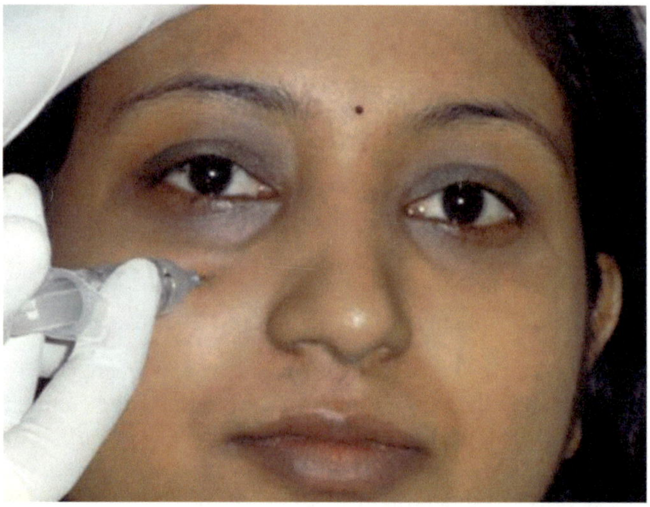

Fig. 4.

A successful Infraorbital nerve block will anesthetize the Infraorbital cheek, the lower palpebral area, the lateral nasal area, and superior labial regions as shown in figure.

3.5 Zygomaticotemporal nerve block

Two uncommon facial local anesthetic blocks are the zygomaticotemporal and zygomaticofacial nerves. This may assist the injection of fillers in facial rhytides on the lateral temporal and lateral canthal areas or in the malar areas. These nerves represent the terminal branches of the zygomatic nerve. The zygomaticotemporal nerve emerges through a foramen located on the anterior wall of the temporal fossa. This foramen is actually behind the lateral orbital rim posterior to the zygoma at the approximate level of the lateral canthus.

To orient for this injection it is necessary to palpate the lateral orbital rim at the level of the frontozygomatic suture (which is frequently palpable). With the index finger in the depression of the posterior lateral aspect of the lateral orbital rim (inferior and posterior to the frontozygomatic suture), the operator places the needle just behind the palpating finger (which is about 1 cm posterior to the frontozygomatic suture). The needle is then 'walked' down the concave posterior wall of the lateral orbital rim to approximate level of the lateral canthus. After aspirating, 1-2mL of 2% lidocaine is injected in this area with a slight pumping action to ensure deposition of the local anesthetic solution at or about the foramen. Again, it is important to hug the back concave wall of the lateral orbital rim with the needle when injecting.

Blocking the zygomaticotemporal nerve causes anesthesia in the area superior to the nerve, including lateral orbital rim and the skin of the temple from above the zygomatic arch to the temporal fusion line.

3.6 Zygomaticofacial nerve block

The zygomaticofacial nerve exits through a foramen (or foramina in some patients) in the inferior lateral portion of the orbital rim at the zygoma. If the surgeon palpates the junction of the inferior lateral portion of the lateral orbital rim, the nerve emerges several millimeters lateral to this point. By palpating this area and injecting just lateral to the finger, this nerve is successfully blocked with 1-2mL of local anesthetic. Blocking this nerve will result in anesthesia of a triangular area from the lateral canthus and the malar region along the zygomatic arch and some skin inferior to this area.

3.7 Mental nerve block

The mental nerve exits the mental foramen on the hemimandible at the base of the root of the second premolar (many patients may be missing a premolar due to orthodontic extraction). The mental foramen is on average 11 mm inferior to the gum line. There is variability with this foramen, but by injecting 2-4 mL of local anesthetic solution about 10 mm inferior to gum line or 15 mm inferior to top of the crown of the second premolar tooth the block is usually successful. In a patient without teeth, the foramen is often times located much higher on the jaw and can sometimes be palpated. This block is performed more superiorly in the denture patient. As stated earlier, the foramen does not need to be entered as a sufficient volume of local anesthetic solution in the general area will be effective. By placing traction on the lip and pulling it away from the jaw, the labial branches of the mental nerve can be seen traversing through the thin mucosa in some patients. The mental nerve gives off labial branches to the lip and chin.

Alternatively, the mental nerve may be blocked through the skin of the cheek with a facial approach, aiming for the same target.

When anesthetized the distribution of numbness will be the unilateral lower lip to the midline and laterally to the mentolabial fold, and in some patients the anterior chin and cheek depending on the individual furcating anatomy of that patient's nerve.

As mentioned earlier, sometimes patients may perceive pain despite bilateral nerve block in the upper or lower lips. When injecting fillers in the lower lip and bilateral mental nerve blocks are not totally effective, a supplemental infiltration of several milliliters of local anesthetics region of the mandibular labial frenulum can assist the block.

Anesthesia for aesthetic lip augmentation[17]

Although in theory a bilateral Infraorbital block should anesthetize the entire upper lip, some patients may still perceive pain for various anatomic (or sometimes psychological) reasons. It is recommended that the injection of 1.0mL of local anesthetic solution in the maxillary labial frenum. This can also be performed in the lower lip labial frenum area to augment bilateral mental blocks.

3.8 Digital nerve block[9]

This is commonly performed nerve block by dermatosurgeons for nail surgeries, acral vitiligo correction, multiple verrucae on fingers, etc.

Each digit is innervated by two dorsal and two ventral branches of nerve as follows:

- Fingers - Radial and ulnar nerves on dorsal surface.
  Median and ulnar nerve on palmar surface
- Toes - Peroneal nerve on dorsal surface.
  Tibial nerve on planter surface.
  Rarely, Saphenous nerve on dorsal aspect of great toe.

Two methods exist for achieving a digital block viz. ring block and metacarpal/metatarsal head technique (anesthetizing the nerves before they enter the digits). Ring block is more commonly used in day to day practice.

Ring block

The 0.5-1 mL of local anesthetic (without adrenaline) is injected with the help of 26 gauge ½ inch needle at the dorsolateral margin of the desired digit at the level of webspace. The needle is advanced further across the dorsal aspect of the digit and the anesthetic solution injected in superficial (subcutaneous) and then deep plane (close to the bone). It is then withdrawn up to the insertion point and rerouted along the palmar surface in a similar manner and after depositing 0.5-1mL, the needle is completely removed. The hand is turned over and needle inserted at the palmar medial surface at level of webspace of the same digit. It is pushed across laterally and solution injected, withdrawn to insertion point, redirected medially to complete the block.

Metacarpal/metatarsal head technique

The needle is introduced in the space between the heads of the metacarpals / metatarsals, proximal to the webspace and perpendicular to skin. It is advanced in a similar direction towards the palmar / plantar aspect of the hand/foot, till it reaches the subcutaneous level here.

The local anesthetic solution is then injected thus blocking the digital nerves at the level before they enter the digit. The needle is withdrawn and the procedure repeated on the other side of the respective metacarpal/metatarsal head.

Since the blood supply to digits is by terminal arteries, adrenaline should not be mixed with local anesthetic. The volume injected to produce block should not exceed 8mL as larger volume can produce mechanical compression on vasculature results in ischemia and digital necrosis.

Sometimes, the anesthesia achieved is unsatisfactory; the reason for this could be failure to infiltrate the local anesthetic close to bone, where nerve lies; or failure to anesthetize adequate length of the nerve. Both causes can be avoided by using higher concentration solutions.

Reducing the pain of local anesthesia[10]

The introduction of needle and infiltration of anesthetic are many times very painful and may provoke intense anxiety and can lead to an unpleasant surgical experience for the patient.

The pain experienced during the administration of local anesthetics may be attributed to the needle puncture of the skin, tissue irritation from the solution, and tissue distention from the infiltration.

To minimize pain physician should be reassuring, distracting patients through conversation or slightly vibrating the skin may decrease their perception of pain. For extremely anxious patients, mild sedation with a benzodiazepine may be helpful.

a. Reducing the needle prick pain[18]
   - Explanation of procedure,
   - Use of mild sedation
   - Use of topical anesthetic cream can be helpful to minimize pain.
   - Use of small diameter needle can be less painful compare to larger diameter needle.
   - Longer needle should be used when anesthetizing large areas to avoid multiple pricks
   - Use of long acting local anesthetic helps to avoid repeated pricks if procedure is more time taking.
   - Slow introduction of needle, introduction of needle through accentuated pore (on face), reinsert needle in an area already anesthetized are other way to reduce the pain associated with needle prick.

b. Reducing the pain associated with tissue distension
   Slow injection of anesthetic solution, only required amount to be injected, inject into subcutaneous fat, use of field block, being injecting the drug proximally and advanced distally (produce anesthesia distal to needle tip reducing the pain of advancing injection needle).

c. Reducing the pain due to tissue irritation
   The tissue irritation from local anesthetics is primarily due to the acidity of the anesthetic solution. The anesthetics are acidified to increase their solubility, as well as their chemical stability. To decrease irritation produced by local anesthetics, the solution may be buffered through several means:
   - Mix lidocaine with adrenaline with plain lidocaine in equal part.
   - Mixed plain lidocaine (10 mL) with adrenaline (0.1mL). The subsequent solution is lidocaine with adrenaline, but at same pH as plain lidocaine.
   - Add sodium bicarbonate to the anesthetic solution (lidocaine with adrenaline: sodium bicarbonate in 10:1) to increase the pH of local anesthetics to near tissue fluid levels.[19]

4. Tumescent anesthesia[20]

This is a technique of local anesthesia which involves the subcutaneous injection of large volumes of dilute LA in combination with adrenaline and other agents is used for dermabrasion, skin grafting, rhinophyma correction, liposuction and hair transplant procedures, most common being liposuction. The plasma concentrations may peak more than 8-12 hours after infusion. Clinicians are advised to exercise great caution in administering additional local anesthesia by infiltration or other routes for at least 12-18 hours following the use of this technique.

4.1 Tumescent fluid – Composition[21]

Normal Saline 1000 cc
Lidocaine (2%) 50 cc
Adrealine (1:1000) 1 cc
Sodium bicarbonate (8.4%) 10 cc
Effective concentration of lidocaine - 0.1%

(Safe up to 55 mg/kg, according to the American Academy of Dermatology guidelines of care for liposuction.)

4.2 Advantages[20,21]

1. The injection is almost painless as it is placed subcutaneously, where the lax tissue is easily distensible
2. It pushes up or stretches the skin and the area to be operated and provides a cushioning effect to deeper structures, so less chance of their damage.
3. Provides very good hemostasis due to large volume of anesthetic compresses the subcutaneous vasculature.
4. It causes hydrodissection at subcutaneous layer and provide safer plane for dissection like in donor strip harvesting in hair transplantation, due to volume of anesthetic injected and also helps to preserve the dermal tissue architecture since injection is placed at deeper level.
5. Smaller quantity of actual anesthetic agent is required for desire action which reduces the possibility of systemic side effects.
6. Prolonged area of several hours' duration occurs as a result of a reservoir effect of local anesthetic.
7. The addition of adrenaline increases the duration of action[5], while sodium bicarbonate helps to adjust the pH of the formulation to a level very close to that of the tissue fluid, which reduces the tissue irritation and pain during the injection of Tumescence anesthesia.
8. Elimination of general anesthesia, hospital operating facilities, and hospital overnight stays also result in a favorable impact on costs when this technique is employed.

4.3 Disadvantages[20]

1. Since the prepared solution is placed subcutaneously, there is more diffusion in this highly distensible compartment and faster absorption through this vascular tissue.
2. Onset of anesthetic action takes 10-15 minutes due to time taken to penetrate the dermal nerves from deeper plane.

4.4 Calculation of maximal tumescent technique lidocaine dose for 70 kg liposuction patient

(55mg/kg)(80kg) = 4400 mg
If 0.1% lidocaine solution is used, then
(4400 mg)/(1mg/L) = 4.400 L
4400 mL of 0.1% solution

4.5 Tumescence infiltration technique

Tumescent fluid is infiltrated in tissue either by a syringe with needle or by infusion canula.

Skin is gently numbed by infiltration of same tumescent solution at places of anticipated adits. Small access openings are made to insert infusion canula attached either to a lure locked syringe or infusion pump. Tumescent fluid in infiltrated till the skin shows pallor. Rate of infusion should be slow to avoid discomfort due to rapid stretching of skin.

Tumescence solutions: concentration, volume, used for various body areas[21]

Area	volume of tumescent Solution ml	Lidocaine (mg/L)	Lidocaine (mg)
Jowels	25-75	1250	30-95
Chin and Neck	50-150	1250	60-190
Male breast	400-1400	1250	500-1750
Upper arms	500-1200	1000	500-1200
Male flanks	500-1100	1000	500-1100
Waist	400-1000	1000	400-1000
Hips	600-1200	750	450-1080
Abdomen, upper	500-1200	1000	500-1200
Abdomen, lower	600-1500	1000	600-1500
Medial thighs	800-1500	750	600-1125
Lateral thighs	400-1300	750	300-975
Knees	200-400	750	150-300

Discomfort during the infusion may be due to[21]

- Too high infusion rate - decrease the rate
- Advancing an infusing cannula too rapidly- consider slower advancement, consider needle infusion, or initiating infusion with needle prior to using infusion cannula

- Skin surface inadequately numbed - re numb the skin.

Local Anesthesia in Hair Transplantation[22]

- Anesthesia for strip removal
  - Infiltration with lidocaine 1cm lower than lower incision line
  - Tumescent fluid infiltration
- Anesthesia in frontal (donor) area
  - Nerve blocks for supra-orbital and supratrochlear
  - Tumescent fluid infiltration
- Anesthesia for FUE donor site
  - Field block
  - Tumescent fluid infiltration

5. Non pharmacological anesthesia

a. Hypnosis, talkasthesia

Many patients may be benefited just by soothing verbal and tactile reinforcement from doctor as well as family members. This works on principle of hypnosis as a tool to enhance the patient's tolerance level. The patient is asked to relax and be calm. Sometimes physician can ask the patient to concentrate on breathing - slow steady inspiration and expiration to the count of 'one-the-three'. - This maneuver helps the majority of the patient to relax and calm. Holding the patient's hand, with or without gentle stroking, is also a calming preocedure.[23]

b. Vibration anesthesia[24]

Vibration has been used for many years to reduce pain in disciplines such as dentistry and physiotherapy, and is now becoming recognized as a simple, safe and effective form of anesthesia in dermatology. Vibration anesthesia can be explained by the 'gate theory of pain control'.[25] populazied by Melzack and Wall in the 1960s. Noxious nerve impulses evoked by injuries are influenced in the spinal cord by other nerve cells that act like gates, either preventing the impulses from getting through, or facilitating their passage. Without vibratory modulation, noxious impulses are carried through small C fibers uninhibited through a 'gate' in the spinal cord that ultimately sends the signal to the brain. When applied simultaneously, vibratory stimulation excites large A fibers, which activates inhibitory interneurons at the gate and mitigates the perception of pain in the brain.

Any vibratory massager can be used to produce the vibratory stimulation. A study has shown that pain sensitivity gradually declines as vibration amplitude increases, but no specific frequency is more effective in interference with nociception. The vibratory massager should be applied approximately 2-3 seconds prior to the injection or laser application and 1-2 cm from the site, and continue throughout the procedure.

c. Cooling[26,27]

Cooling can be achieved using sprays, cold air, ice, ice packs, and gels. Cooling can reduce the discomfort of many procedures. Both pain and temperature sensation travel in the same nerve pathway. If this nerve pathway is overloaded by the cold sensation, pain is less likely to be felt in the same area.

Refrigerant spray: It is a form of cryoanesthesia, which works on 'gate theory' of pain control.[25] It is a spray containing ethyl chloride or dichlorotetrafluroethane. The refrigerant is sprayed for 2-5 seconds, depending upon the distance from the skin until a white frost is seen and then immediately the short procedure has to be carried out

5.1 Cooling methods for various lasers[28]

Cooling in laser procedures acts not only as numbing agent but a epidermal protector. Following are various ways to cool epidermis while achieving changes in deeper part of skin.

- Icing before laser
- Cool air flow (Zimmer Cryo)
- DCD spray
- Sapphire tip contact cooling
- Metal tip contact cooling
- Cool gel

5.2 Role of anesthesia in outcome of aesthetic procedure:

Anesthesia in aesthetic procedures has not only a functional role but also has a great psychological impact on perception of the procedure by the patient. Successful anesthesia and analgesia makes the aesthetic procedure a pleasant experience for the patients and encourage them to go for such repeated procedures.

6. Summary

Local anesthesia makes cosmetic procedures not only appealing but cost effective also by making them day care ones. A topical anesthetic cream with occlusion is most common technique of local anesthesia. Field block is achieved by infiltration of LA in and around area to be treated. It is modified to target an innervating nerve trunk by various nerve blocks. Tumescent local anesthesia is a state of art modification of LA to anesthetize a very large volume of tissue for prolonged period without significant adverse effects. Mastering the art and science of local anesthesia is very much essential in successful outcome of aesthetic procedures.

7. References

[1] Strichartz GR. Neural physiology and local anesthetic action. In: Cousins MJ, Bridenbaugh PO, eds. Neural blockade in clinical anesthesia and management of pain. Philadelphia: JB Lippincott, 1988:25–45.
[2] Auletta MJ. Local anesthesia for dermatologic surgery. Semin Dermatol 1994;13:35–42.
[3] Tucker GT, Mather LE. Properties, absorption, and deposition of local anesthetic agents. In: Cousins MJ, Bridenbaugh PO, eds. Neural blockade in clinical anesthesia and management of pain. Philadelphia: JB Lippincott, 1988:47–110.
[4] Auletta MJ, Grekin RC. Local anesthesia for dermatologic surgery. New York: Churchill Livingstone, 1991:1–40.
[5] Satoskar RS, Bhandarkar SD: Pharmacology and Pharmacotherapeutics 12th edn., Bombay: Popular Prakashan Pvt. Ltd. 1992; 189-194.

[6] Covino BG, Vassallo HG. Local anesthetics: mechanisms of action and clinical use. New York: Grune & Stratton, 1976:1–148.
[7] Dzubow LM. The interaction between propranolol and epinephrine as observed in patients undergoing Moh's surgery. J Am Acad Dermatol 1986;15:71–5.
[8] Glinert RJ, Zachary CB. Local anesthesia allergy. J Dermatol Surg Oncol 1991;17:491–6.
[9] Auletta Mj, Grekin RC: Clinical application of local anesthesia. Local Aneshtesia for Dermatologic Surgery 1st edn., New York: Churchill Livingstone 1991;41-78
[10] Auletta Mj, Grekin RC: Tricks to make the delivery of local anesthesia less painful. Local anesthesia for Dermatologic Surgery 1st edn., New York: Churchill Livingstone 1991; 79-84.
[11] Green SS. Iontophoresis as a tool for anesthesia in dermatology surgery: an overview. Dermatol Surg 2001; 27:1027-30
[12] Baron Elma, Harris Lisbeth, Redpath William S et al. Laser assisted penetration of topical anesthetics in adults. Arch Dermatol 2003; 139:1288-90
[13] Hædersdal, M., Sakamoto, F. H., Farinelli, W. A., Doukas, A. G., Tam, J. and Anderson, R. R. (2010), Fractional CO_2 laser-assisted drug delivery. Lasers in Surgery and Medicine, 42: 113–122.
[14] Friedman PM., Mafong E, Friedman E et al. Topical anesthetic update: Emla and beyond. Dermatol Surg 2001; 27:1019-26.
[15] Splinter W.M, 'Needle-Free' Delivery of Local Anesthesia: A Valuable Option in Pediatrics. Pediatric Drugs 2002; 4: 349-52.
[16] Banga AK, Bose S, Ghosh TK. Iontophoresis and electroporation: comparisons and contrasts, International Journal of Pharmaceutics. 1999; 179(2): 1-19
[17] Carruthers J, Carruthers A. (Eds). *Soft Tissue Augmentation,*New Delhi:Elsevier 2006, 155-159.
[18] Arndt KA, Burton C, Noe JM. Minimizing the pain of local anesthesia. Plast Reconstr Surg 1993;72:676-9.
[19] Skidmore RA, Patterson JD, Tomsick RS. Local anesthetics. Dermatol Surg 1996;22:511-22.
[20] Klein JA: Anesthesia for liposuction in dermatologic surgery. J Derm Surg Oncol 1988; 14: 1124-32.
[21] William Hanke C, Sattler G (Eds). *Liposuction.* New Delhi:Elsevier 2007; 21-32.
[22] Seager DJ, Simmons C. Local Anesthesia in Hair Transplantation. Dermatologic Surgery. 2002; 28: 320–328.
[23] Spiegel H, Spiegel D. Trance and treatment clinical use of hypnosis. New York: Basic Books; 1978
[24] Smith KC, Comite SL, Balasubramanian S. Vibration anesthesia: A noninvasive method of reducing discomfort prior to dermatologic procedures. Dermatology Online Journal 10 (2): 1
[25] Melzack R, Wall PD. Pain mechanisms: a new theory. Science. 1965 Nov 19;150(699):971-9.
[26] Chan HH, Lam LK, Wong DS, Wei WI. Role of skin cooling in improving patient tolerability of Q-switched Alexandrite (QS Alex) laser in nevus of Ota treatment. Lasers Surg Med. 2003;32(2):148-51
[27] Kauvar AN, Frew KE, Friedman PM, Geronemus RG. Cooling gel improves pulsed KTP laser treatment of facial telangiectasia. Lasers Surg Med. 2002;30(2):149-53.
[28] Nanni CA, Alster TS. Laser-assisted hair removal: Side effects of Q-switched Nd:YAG, long-pulsed ruby, and alexandrite lasers. J Am Acad Dermatol. 1999;41:165-71.

3

Repair of Incisional Hernias of the Midline Under Local Anesthesia in an Ambulatory Basis

Alberto F. Acevedo
Hernia Center, Reference Health Center "Cordillera", Santiago
Universidad de Chile, Medicine Faculty, Surgical Department
Salvador Hospital, Santiago
Chile

1. Introduction

1.1 General considerations

1. The selection of patients is important when performing this rather big surgical procedures with local anesthesia. Those who prefer general or regional anesthesia and patients with adverse reactions to LA should be excluded, as well as patients with psychological and psiquiatric conditions.
2. An experienced surgeon in the use of local anesthesia will not only perform a better anesthesia but will positively influence his patient during the intervention. The surgeon-patient relationship is relevant in these cases.
3. The surgeon should be experienced in the management of the abdominal wall in order to realize a technically adequate procedure in a short time, with a careful and delicate management of tissues.
4. In these midline incisional hernias the hole length of the scar should be excised and the midline explored because of the multisacularity condition of these defects (7).
5. New surgical techniques to be used under local anesthesia should be ideally be developed and submitted to clinical tests in specialized centers, by experts and tested scientifically. Our hernia center gathers all these conditions (8).

1.2 Our experience

Patients with hernial-sacs smaller as 15cm and a width of the hernial-ring smaller as 4cm. were accepted in our program to be operated in an ambulatory basis, under local anesthesia Fig. 1.

Patients accomplishing the social, financial, psychological and health conditions requirable for these procedures signed an informed consensus and in general accepted gladly to be incorporated to the program (8).

Obesity with a BMI up to 45 and compensated diabetes mellitus were not considered a motive for exclusion of patients from the program

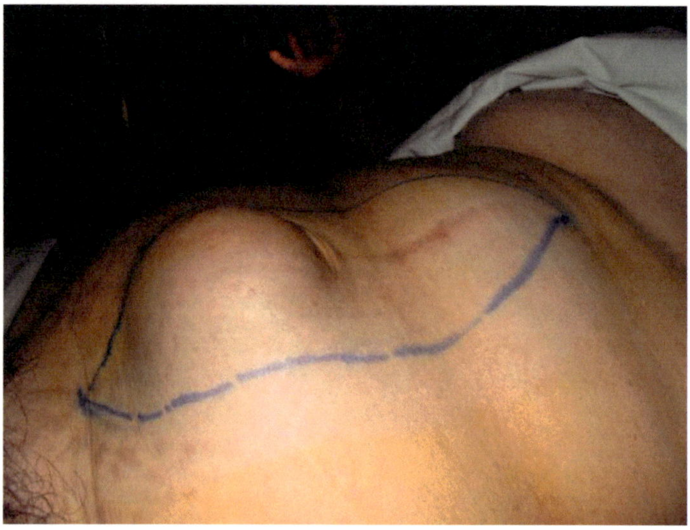

Fig. 1. Incisonal hernia of the midline and umbilical hernia. The blue line shows the skin incision.

1.3 Anesthesia

The day of surgery patents were allowed to drink water or tea, but no solid meals. Medications for chronic conditions as diabetes mellitus and hypertension were not suspended. Patients got there skin prepared as usual, entered the op room and were placed supine at the operation table with a light head down tilt. The anesthetist applied sedation and keeped control of vital signs, ECG, O2 and CO2.

Antiseptic preparation of the skin and local anesthesia was applied before the preparation of the operation field in order to obtain a deeper anesthesia.

For theses big operation fields we performed local anesthesia by means of a quite diluted Lidocain solution (0,3 - 0,5%), alkalinized with sodium bicarbonate and with adrenalin addition.

It's recommendable that the surgeon traces a line over the skin lozenge to be excised over the hernial sac, because it's going to exceed as the underlying rectus sheaths are approached to each other to build a new "linea alba". In lean patients the skin excision should be narrower as in obese (Fig 1).

1.4 Summary of local anesthesia repair

1. Subcuticular injection of anesthetic. It's performed in the whole length of the skin incision (40 - 60ml).
2. Infiltration of the subcutaneous tissue in all the length of the surgical wound (60 - 100ml).
3. Infiltration of the rectus muscle through the aponeurosis (Fig. 2).The surgeon makes the skin incision down to the rectus sheath. Deposits of 2 - 3ml Lidocain solution should be realized each 2 - 3cm, in al the length of the wound at both sides (30 - 40ml).

4. The skin and subcutaneous tissue lozenge is excised together. Small amounts of anesthesia may be necessary at the point where the nerves perforate the rectus Sheath to achieve the skin. (10 - 20ml)
5. At this point the hernial sacs are exposed and the surgeon can recognize its number and the width of the hernial rings.
6. The Double Invaginating Isotensional Repair (DIIR) technique proposed makes it unnecessary to perform an incision in the "linea alba". The sacs are simply individually reduced as the first isotensional suture is performed (Fig. 4 - a).
7. While the second and third suture line of the DIIR are performed (Fig. 4 - b, c), it is possible that further Lidocain deposits in the rectus muscle are needed (10 - 20ml).
8. This surgery needs sedation performed by the anesthetist whose presence in the operation theatre is mandatory.

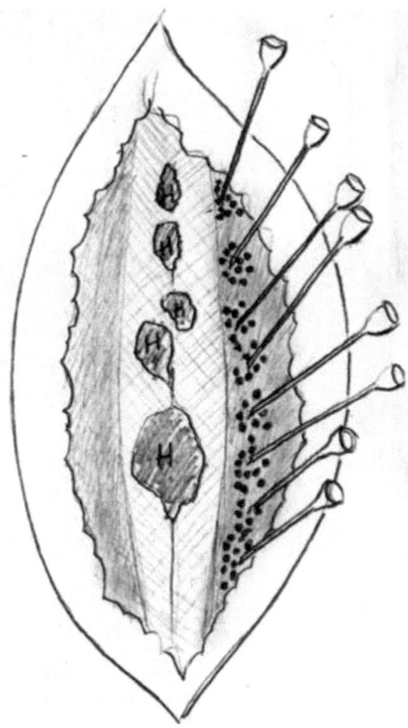

Fig. 2. Deposits of local anestheticum in the rectus muscle.

1.5 Concomitant umbilical, epigastric hernia and middle line diastases repair

These pathologies may coexist with the incisional hernia and can be simultaneously treated with this technique under local anesthesia (9). In these cases it is necessary to act up on the umbilicus which in small defects can be preserved. In bigger ones it is better to extirpate it and build a new one with a skin plastic.

In this case local anesthesia and skin incision should be prolonged some 3 - 4cm under the umbilicus. The umbilical and epigastric hernial sacs are treated similarly as the incisional hernia ones (Figs. 1,3).

1.6 Intraoperative monitoring

Through the operation the anesthesia assistant nurse stays by the patient attending his necessities and maintaining his attention away from the operative procedure. She kips a written report of the evolution of the vital signs, well being of the patients, as well of the adverse reactions and their treatment.

The stress reaction during local anesthesia varies considerably from patient to patient and manifests it's self through the vital signs (hypertension, tachycardia) and through nervousness and restlessness that should be managed by the anesthetist with the required pharmacological support.

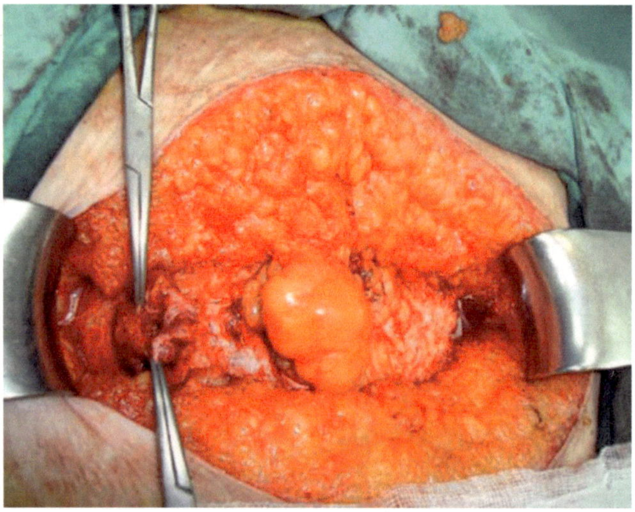

Fig. 3. Multisacular incisional hernia of the midline. The umbilical hernia has bin already reduced.

1.7 Postoperative care

The surgical wound is dressed and covered by an elastic girdle. Immediately after the operation the patient sits in the operation table, stays up and walks some 10 meters to the postoperative care station where he sits in a comfortable armchair. At this point the anesthetist and the postoperative care nurse take care of the patient.

At this stage the patient is allowed to take a breakfast in the company of a family member. As a precaution a saline vein-infusion is maintained during this period.

After an observation time of 2 - 4hours the patient dresses and is carried in a wheel chair to the CRS entry to be translated to his home.

Detailed indications are provided to the patient and his family as well as a telephone number in order to stay in touch with the CRS Hernia Center. Bed rest is restricted and moving, walking and activities at home are enhanced.

The patient is appointed to a personal control at the CRS the day after the operation where the wound is inspected and the evolution kept under carful observation. Controls are made a week and a month after the intervention.

2. Operative technique

Consideration should be paid to the fact that multisacularity is a frequent condition in theses hernias (Fig. 3). Among our patients it affects 83% if the hernias of the midline (Table 1). This fact makes it imperative to explore the scar in all its length (6).

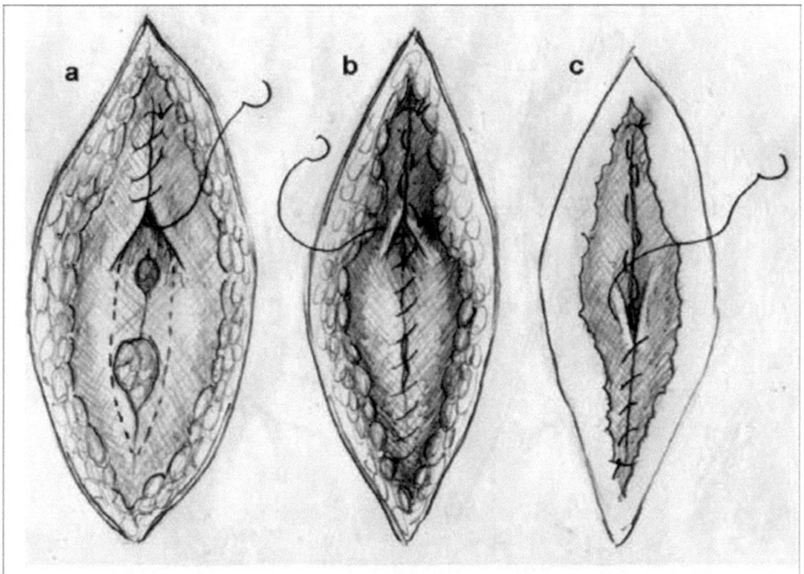

Fig. 4. a.- The midline defect is closed by means of an isotensional suture in al the length of the xifo-umbilical midline; b.- first row of invaginating suture; c.- second row of invaginating suture.

We considered the performance of tissue repair by means of an original technique developed in our Hernia Center (9). This technique pursue a reconstruction of the "linea alba" by means of an isotensional repair followed by a double invaginating suture (DIIR) (Fig 3).

This tissue technique is performed if the hernial ring borders can be sutured without tension (usually in defects not wider as 3cm). In wider defects a flat Prolene mesh patch was installed in a sub-lay position and fixed to the aponeurosis with transfixing Prolene sutures.

In a prospective study performed in these patients(10) we could demonstrate that the drainage can be replaced with slowly absorbable interrupted subcutaneous sutures anchored to the aponeurosis (10) (Fig. 5, 6).

Number of hernial sacs	n patients	%
1	44	17
2	129	49.5
3	47	18.1
4 or more	40	15.4
Total	260	100

Table 1. Multisacularity of incisional hernias of the midline

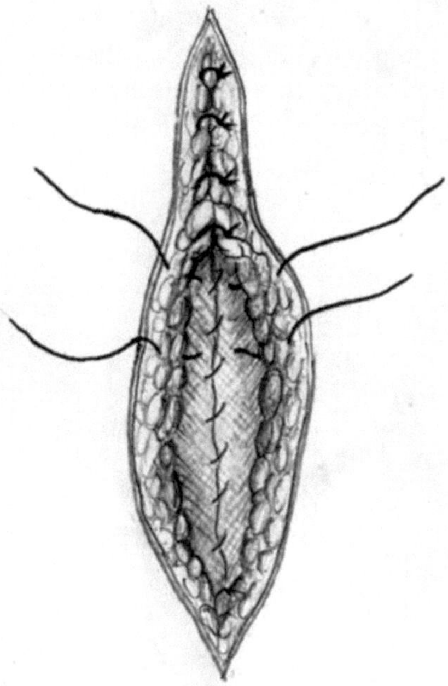

Fig. 5. Schematic representation of the subcutaneous anchored suture

The skin is closed with an intradermal continuous suture (Fig. 7)

3. Clinical experience

The preoperative, operative and postoperative evolution of our patients was kept in the data base of the CRS Hernia Center constructed with the software of epidemiologic calculus "Epi Info".

We give account of a study performed recently (9) on 260 patients with incisional hernias of the midline. At first we started a controlled clinical trial between mesh and tissue repair of midline incisional hernias, but this study developed with time to an observational one because of the obvious benefits obtained with the tissue repair performed with the DIIS. A mesh was installed in 71 patients, while 189 cases received a DIIR (Tables 2, 3).

Characteristics and associated pathologies were similar in patients treated with mesh and tissue repair.

This patients-series is composed by 207 women and 53 men with a middle age of 54 +/- 8,6 years. Obesity (BMI>30) was present in 51.2% of the patients, being observed in a significantly higher proportion among women (P<0.021).

A first repair of the incisional hernia was performed in 86% of the patients; a recurrent hernia was present in the rest.

The hernial sac was bigger as 10 cm in 64% of patients and smaller in the rest. Obese patients showed a significantly higher proportion of sacs bigger as 10cm (P<0,03).

The number of sacs observed in our series varies considerably (Table 1).

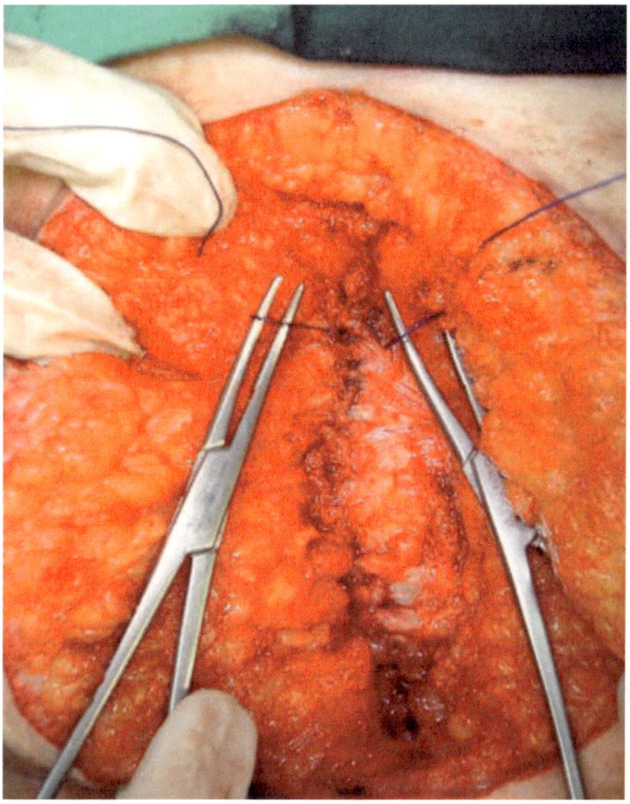

Fig. 6. Subcutaneous anchored suture.

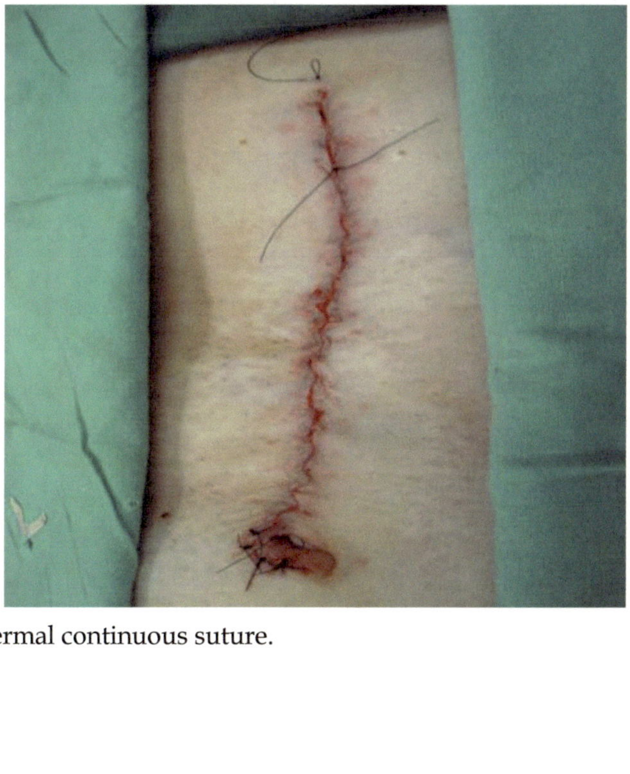

Fig. 7. Skin intradermal continuous suture.

YEARS	Mesh (%)	Tissue (%)
1998 - 2000	25 (62.5)	15 (37.5)
2001 - 2003	20 (27)	54 (73)
2004 - 2006	19 (20.7)	73 (79.3)
2007 - 2009	7 (7.9)	47 (82.1)
TOTAL	71	189

Table 2. Distribution of our patients in the years

TECHNIQUES	n
Mesh	71
DIIS	160
Simple suture	29
TOTAL	260

Table 3. Techniques performed in our series

3.1 Intraoperative evolution (Table 4)

Care was paid to follow the technique previously described.

Under theses circumstances the intraoperative pain and discomfort referred by the patients was comparable with the one observed in the repair of huge and complex inguinal hernias.

Although we have performed some interventions in patients with xifo-pubic incisional hernias, a spinal anesthesia is better option in theses cases. We would recommend local anesthesia only when the general condition of the patient demands it.

The presence of the anesthetist is mandatory in these procedures, especially in obese patients. Aside from troubles derived from the surgery it's self, the surgery lasts longer in obese patients that feel uncomfortable in a supine position at the operation table.

3.2 Postoperative evolution (Table 4)

The first control was realized 24 hours after the operation. Our purpose was to control the mobility of patients and to have a look to the performance of daily activities at home. Motility, respiratory and digestive tract functions were evaluated.

At this early stage of the evolution, abdominal pain was the principal complaint of patients, understandable because of the traction of the flat muscles of the abdominal wall upon the suture in the midline. It decreases after the third day, especially in patients that remain active.

The postoperative analgesia in incisional herniorrhaphy is a very important issue. Every group of surgeons will have its one approach to this fundamental point of surgical treatment.

We mind that patients should be informed that pain is the natural consequence of surgery. A patient that has been prepared to his postoperative evolution will have a better control and management of pain the days after surgery.

We are recommending Ketoprofen 100mg each 12 hours and Paracetamol 500mg each 8 hours for the first 3 or 4 days after surgery.

At the thirtieth day it is possible to obtain a more realistic impression of the patient over his surgical treatment. Impressive is the high proportion of patients being very satisfied with the herniorrhaphy performed under local anesthesia in an ambulatory basis.

Infections were present in mesh and tissue techniques that were treated ambulatory with drainage and antibiotics. The two infected prosthetic repairs healed without removal of the mesh.

Information	mesh	tissue	p-value
Intraopertive			
Op duration minutes (St)	73 (12)	49 (18)	<0,02
Pain (VAS)	2,1 (0,4)	2,2 (0,3)	ns
Postoperative (24hours)			
Pain (VAS < 3)	79%	71%	<0,04
Satisfaction (VAS>7)	97%	87%	<0,032
Recommend this surgery	89.2%	83%	ns
Nausea	4,2%	3,8%	ns
Bed rest the first day	9,6%	12,1%	ns
Self sufficiency at home	76%	83,6%	ns
Alimentary intolerance	2,1%	3,2%	ns
Urine retention	0,4%	1,2%	ns
Emergency unit attendance	1,2%	0	ns
Re-admittance	0,2%	0	ns
Postoperative (30 days)			
Pain (VAS <3)	98,2%	97,1%	ns
Satisfaction (VAS>7)	98.2%	96,5%	ns
Infection	3,6	3,2	ns
Hematomas	0	1,2	ns

Table 4. Intra and postoperative follow-up of the patients

3.3 Long time follow-up

In a study published 2009 we gave account of a follow-up performed in 85% of 116 patients treated with the DIIR and 23 with sub-lay mesh hernioplasty (10). Seventeen DIIS and 3 mesh hernioplasty patients were not available for this study for different reasons. The study performed following the strict criteria proposed by Israelsson (11).

Patients treated with prosthetic and tissue repair were personally controlled by a staff member after a follow-up period of 6 (2,8 - 8) years. The recurrence rate was 12% for the mesh repairs and of 6% for the DIIR.

A high proportion of patients was satisfied or highly satisfied with ambulatory surgery under local anesthesia (98%) and would recommend it. The two unsatisfied patients had pain in the lateral abdomen with restriction of usual activities.

4. Final commentary

A surgeon with experience in abdominal wall surgery and in the performance of local anesthesia is imperative for the success in the treatment of these more complex hernias of the abdominal wall under local anesthesia.

The tissue repair under local anesthesia for small size incisional hernias with the proposed DIIR technique has become the standard treatment for these patients. It simplifies and shortens the surgical repair of these hernias and makes possible its realization in an ambulatory basis.

Surgical complications are seldom and the acceptance of patients operated in our Centrum has proven to be very good.

5. References

[1] Chevrel JP, Rath AM. Classification of incisional hernias of the abdominal wall. Hernia 2000; 4: 7 - 11

[2] Herszage L. Indication and limitations of suture closure. Significance of relaxing incisions. In Schumpelick V, Kingsnorth AM. Incisional hernia. Springer Verlag, Berlin Heildelberg, 1999, pp279 - 286

[3] Muysoms FE, Miserez M, Berrevoet F, Campanelli G, Champault GG, Chelala E, et al. Classification of primary and incisional abdominal wall hernias. Hernia 2009; 13: 407 - 14

[4] Flament JB, Rives J. Major incisional hernias. In Chevrel JP, hernias and surgery of the abdominal wall. Springer Verlag, Berlin, 1998, pp128 - 158

[5] Stoppa RE. The treatment of complicated groin and incisional hernias. World J Surg 1989;13: 545 554

[6] Wantz GE. Incisional hernioplasty with Mersilene. Surg Gynecol Obstet 1991; 172: 129 - 137

[7] Acevedo A. Multisacularidad de las eventraciones de la línea media. Cuaderno de resúmenes del LXXVII Congreso Chileno de Cirugía, Pucón, 2004

[8] Acevedo A, Viterbo A, Bravo J, Dellepiane V. Eventraciones, cirugía ambulatoria con anestesia local. Rev Chil Cir 2006; 58: 354 - 358

[9] Acevedo A, Lombardi J, Leon J, López J, Schultz E, Dellepiane V. Eventraciones. Reconstrucción plástica xe la línea alba mediante doble sutura invaginante isotensional (DSII). Rev Chil Cir. 2009; 61: 339 - 344

[10] Acevedo A, Viterbo A, Cápona R, Dellepaine V. Prescindencia de drenaje en la eventrorrafia ambulatoria. Rev Chil Cir. 2008; 60: 291 - 296

[11] Israelsson LA, Smedberg S, Montgomery A, Nordin P, Spangen L. Incisional hernia repair in Sweden 2002. Hernia 2006; 10: 256 - 261

Urological Surgical Procedures Under Local Anesthesia

M. Hammad Ather[1], Ammara Mushtaq[2] and M. Nasir Sulaiman[1]
[1]Dept of Surgery, Aga Khan University
[2]Dow University of Health Sciences
Pakistan

1. Introduction

Surgical procedures under local anesthesia provide unique advantages. They are associated with less patient anxiety antecedent with the use of general or major regional anesthesia. It is also associated with quicker recovery, less day care recovery room stay and earlier returns to work. It is therefore not surprising that there is considerable interest both among patients and surgeons. The impetus for this has been to maximize anesthetic and postoperative resources by increasing patient turnover in the operating room and discharging patients more efficiently on the same day. Patients with significant co-morbidities, with relative or absolute contra-indication to general or major regional anesthesia can also undergo procedures safely. The use of local anesthesia has continued to expand the ability of urologists to perform a variety of procedures in a safer fashion, particularly in high-risk patients. Most of the local procedures are performed in an operating room setting with a nurse anesthetist in attendance that may administer small amounts of additional intravenous sedation during the procedure. The main goal is to have the patient comfortable during the procedure, but also to be awake and conversant. The local anesthesia techniques vary according to site and procedure. Patient selection is critical for the success of any procedure under local anesthesia. The patient must not be overly anxious and must be willing to accept the surgical technique and anesthesia that is described in detail during the preoperative discussion.

Most of the endourological procedures are done as day cases. Some of these can be performed under local anesthesia. The advantage of using local anesthesia includes performing these in the office. This can potentially decrease the cost and lessen the burden on the operating room and recovery room. Some of the standard procedures currently being done include transrectal guided biopsy, flexible cystoscopy, percutaneous nephrostomy, percutaneous cyst aspiration, renal biopsy, and various scrotal procedures. Some of the other procedures that are being done include optical urethrotomy, rigid cystoscopy, bladder biopsy, ureteroscopy, transurethral incision and resection of the prostate, ureteral meatotomy, and resection of primary and recurrent bladder tumors. More recently transurethral needle ablation of the prostate has also been successfully performed under sedoanalgesia. There are few reports on performing percutaneous nephrolithotomy under local anesthesia for selected patients with renal stones. Other transurethral procedures like laser vaporization have also been performed under sedoanalgesia.

The safety profile of local anesthetic agents is well established, however, there are few rare but serious complications. Local anesthesia is sometimes associated with systemic toxicity. This local anesthetic systemic toxicity (LAST) has been a topic of contemporary interest. Although the exact cause and management of LAST (particularly local anesthetic cardiotoxicity) is unclear, there have been some recommendations. Current data suggests that the LAST cardiotoxicity occurs primarily at sodium channels. Lipid emulsion is a reasonably well-tolerated and effective treatment, and there may be qualitative differences in cardiotoxicity caused by low and high-potency local anesthetics (Wolfe and Butterworth, 2011). Treatment is mostly supportive and includes ventilation; oxygenation, and chest compressions, lipid emulsion therapy should be a primary modality in the treatment of cardiovascular LAST. The use of epinephrine and vasopressin should be tailored and doses should be kept as low as possible while still achieving the desired effects (Wolfe and Butterworth, 2011). Seizure suppression is essential to management, and it is further recommended that an earlier communication with a perfusion team for possible cardiopulmonary bypass (Weinberg, 2010).

This chapter deals with focused literature review on the use of local anesthesia for various urological procedures.

2. Inguino-scrotal procedures

Many inguino-scrotal procedures both in the pediatric and adults can be safely performed under local anesthesia. These procedures include simple inguinal hernia repair, inguinal lymph node biopsy, hydrocelectomy, testicular biopsy, testicular fixation, orchidectomy and scrotal exploration (Magoha, 1998). See table 1

Inguino scrotal procedures	Technique
Hydrocelectomy	Cord block and local infiltration
Vasectomy	Cord block and local infiltration
Varicocelectomy	Local infiltration
Testicular biopsy	Cord block and local infiltration or local infiltration alone
Orchidectomy	Cord block and local infiltration
Orchidopexy, inguinal hernia	Cord block and local infiltration
Circumcision	Penile block and local infiltration

Table 1. Some of the common inguino scrotal procedures and technique of anesthesia

These procedures are performed under local anesthesia using various quantities of local anesthetics with or without adrenaline depending on the procedure. Local anesthesia is in the form of spermatic cord block and/or local infiltration nerve blocks. Generally no premedication is required except for anxious patients. Many authors have studied the safety of local anesthetic agents. Magoha (Magoha, 1998) did not report any complication directly attributed to the anesthetic agent used or the technique of spermatic cord and nerve blocks employed. In his reported work majority (97%) of the patients' were treated as a day case. The additional use of spermatic cord block along with local infiltration with xylocaine ± adrenaline is simple, safe and effective technique that should be used more widely in outpatient urological and general surgical settings in inguino-scrotal surgeries.

In a randomized, double-blind controlled study, in 48 patients undergoing day-case testicular surgery under general anesthesia, Burden and colleagues (Burden et al., 1997) in addition to incision site infiltration gave 22 of these patients 10 mL of 0.5% plain bupivacaine into the spermatic cord at the conclusion of surgery. The visual-analogue pain scores were significantly lower in the immediate recovery period in patients receiving the spermatic-cord block.

2.1 Hydrocelectomy

Collection of fluid in the layers of tunica vaginalis has traditionally been treated by surgery. Use of systemic anesthesia with its attendant risks rarely over weigh the discomfort related with this benign condition. Surgeries under local anesthesia and sclerotherapy have become attractive alternative to hydrocelectomy. Aspiration and sclerotherapy is considered cheaper, less invasive and safe compared to hydrocelectomy. However, the outcomes are inconsistent because of lack of uniformity in methods and sclerosing agents used (Khaniya et al., 2009). In another study Beiko et al. (Beiko et al., 2003) similarly concluded that in the treatment of hydroceles, aspiration and sclerotherapy with sodium tetradecylsulfate represents a minimally invasive approach that is simple, inexpensive, and safe but less effective than hydrocelectomy. Sclerotherapy was used in recurrent cases of hydrocele but nowadays due to allergic reaction to sclerosant substances this procedure is not recommended

Hydrocelectomy under local anesthetic is performed in the day care operating room. Patients are continually monitored for hemodynamic stability EKG, blood pressure and oximeter. Any of the local anesthetic agents can be used for local infiltration into the spermatic cord and the site of incision on the scrotal wall. Surgical techniques range from dissection to scission of the bag until partial eversion, requiring the use of reabsorbable suture and a careful hemostasis to avoid drainage. Marchal and colleagues (Marchal et al., 1993) noted that anesthetics tolerance has been highly satisfactory in 52 patients (94%), good in one patient (2%) and unsatisfactory in two cases (4%). Recorded complications in their series included: severe bradycardia and hypotension in one case (2%), persistent right renoureteral pain in one case (2%), scrotal hematoma in 5 cases (9%) and suture dehiscence in another patient (2%). They concluded that surgical management of vaginal collection with local anesthetics is feasible, and reduces the immediate postoperative period also avoiding morbidity derived from a more aggressive anesthetic technique.

2.2 Vasectomy

Vasectomy is advancement in male contraception method keeping in view the increasing number of unwanted or unplanned pregnancies (Page et al., 2008). In Vasectomy, the vasa deferentia are severed. It is the most effective and the most long-term acting form of male contraception (Shih et al., 2011). This surgical procedure performed under local anesthesia is more reliable than classical condoms and timely withdrawal. It is cost-effective, successful and simple when compared to other modes of contraception.

2.2.1 Techniques

After induction of local anesthesia, the procedure involves exposing the vasa to occlude it. Based on the review of surgical techniques by Labrecque and associates (Labrecque et al., 2004), no-scalpel vasectomy (NSV) had less surgical complications than other incisional techniques. Other approaches to access vas deferens for vasectomy include pinhole or keyhole, lateral incisions and electro-cautery techniques but they are still investigational in nature. However, the technique used to expose the vas does not relate to effectiveness of the procedure, rather it is the ligation method used that affects its success (Sokal and Labrecque, 2009). The effectiveness of vasectomy is mainly gauged by post-vasectomy semen analysis and at times, by the rates of pregnancy (Sokal and Labrecque, 2009). No-scalpel vasectomy provides additional advantage in terms of pain control and recovery. Shih and colleagues in 2010 (Shih et al., 2010) reported outcome in pain control by using a mini-needle technique provides excellent anesthesia for no-scalpel vasectomy. They noted that it compares favorably to the standard vasal block and other anesthetic alternatives with the additional benefit of minimal equipment and less anesthesia.

2.3 Varicocelectomy

Varicocele surgery is most commonly performed for infertility secondary to deranged seminal parameters in men with varicocele. Rarely varicocelectomy is also performed for refractory orchalgia secondary to varicocele not responding to conservative management. It seems that this procedure is not effective. The standard management of varicocele repair is the subject of ongoing controversy. In a comparative study of three surgical methods of varicocele treatment Watanabe and colleagues (Watanabe et al., 2005) compared various minimally invasive method. They compared retroperitoneal high ligation under lumbar anesthesia, laparoscopic ligation under general anesthesia, and subinguinal microscopic ligation under local anesthesia. They concluded that subinguinal microscopic varicocelectomy could be a minimally invasive procedure compared to the other two techniques and a worthy method for treating male infertility due to clinical varicocele. In a metanalysis Cayan and colleagues (Cayan et al., 2009) also concluded that the microsurgical varicocelectomy technique has higher spontaneous pregnancy rates and lower postoperative recurrence and hydrocele formation than conventional varicocelectomy techniques in infertile men. Microscopic subinguinal varicocele ligation can be safely performed under local anesthesia. Local infiltration with 1% lidocaine and additional use of cord block provides satisfactory analgesia during the procedure.

In another work Hsu and colleagues (Hsu et al., 2005) performed high ligation of the internal spermatic vein for treatment of a varicocele testis under a regional block in which a precise injection of 0.8 % lidocaine solution was delivered to involved tissues after exact anatomical references were made. They noted that the procedure is simple, effective, reliable and reproducible, and a safe method with minimal complications. It offers the advantages of more privacy, lower morbidity, with no notable adverse effects resulting from anesthesia, and a more rapid return to regular physical activity with minor complications.

2.4 Testicular biopsy, orchidopexy and orchidectomy

Almost all testicular procedures can be safely performed using local anesthesia. The technique used in most cases includes infiltration of local anesthetic at the site of incision on the testicular wall prior to which local anesthesia is given for blocking of the spermatic cord. This technique provides a highly satisfactory pain control as demonstrated by many studies. Slight variation in which testicular parenchyma and tunical albuginea is blocked in place of spermatic cord has also been described. Fahmy and colleagues (Fahmy et al., 2005) described a simple technique to deliver local anesthetic for percutaneous testis biopsies. With the testis held firmly, a 25 gage needle is used to inject lidocaine, without epinephrine, into the skin and dartos superficial to the testis, then the needle is advanced through the tunica albuginea and 0.5 mL to 1.0 mL of lidocaine is injected directly into the testis. The testis becomes slightly more turgid with the injection. A percutaneous biopsy is then immediately performed. The investigators (Fahmy et al., 2005) concluded that intra-testicular lidocaine appears to be a simple, rapid and safe method to provide anesthesia for a percutaneous testis biopsy.

Orchidectomy is most commonly performed as a method of hormonal ablation in advanced prostate cancer. It is either performed as total or subcapsular techniques. In a comparison of the two techniques Roosen and colleagues (Roosen et al., 2005) noted that subcapsular orchiectomy is associated with significantly fewer postoperative complications than total orchidectomy. Desmond and colleagues (Desmond et al., 1988) operated on 100 patients with carcinoma of the prostate by bilateral subcapsular orchidectomy under local anesthesia over a 5-year period. They noted that the procedure is simple, effective and well tolerated by the patients. Inguinal orchidectomy performed for testicular cancer can also be similarly performed under local infiltration and cord block. However, due to inadequate muscle relaxation this technique is not an appropriate procedure for both patient and surgeon.

Pediatric inguino-scrotal procedures like circumcision, inguinal hernia and orchidopexy can be safely performed with caudal block. In an open study by Taylor and colleagues (Taylor et al., 2003) designed to assess the efficacy and safety of 0.25% levobupivacaine administered as a caudal injection at a dose of 2 $mg \cdot kg^{-1}$ to 49 pediatric patients aged less than 2 years old undergoing circumcision (group 1), or hernia repair or orchidopexy (group 2). They noted that adequate analgesia (an increase of <20% in pulse or respiratory rate compared with baseline and an absence of gross movement on application of surgical stimulus) was achieved in 43/48 patients evaluable for efficacy (89.6%). All 22 patients in the circumcision group had adequate analgesia, and two of these patients did not require additional analgesics.

In an interesting work by Kiesling et al. (Kiesling et al., 1984) of using spermatic cord block and manual reduction as a primary treatment for spermatic cord torsion. A total of 16 consecutive cases of acute torsion of the spermatic cord less than 24 hours in duration are presented. All patients were diagnosed and treated initially by spermatic cord blockade and attempted manual detorsion. Of the 16 patients, 15 underwent successful detorsion under local anesthesia. All patients underwent subsequent bilateral orchidopexy. Testicular salvage was 93 per cent in those patients who underwent successful detorsion by manipulation. In complicated torsion cases it is emphasized that the scrotum should be opened and after detorsionizing the testis , cord should be fixed.

3. Penile procedures

Many penile procedures like penile prostheses implantation, modified Nesbit procedure, dorsal slit (Fig 1), venous surgery, venous patches, and arterial revascularization can be safely performed under pure local anesthesia (Hsu et al., 2007).

Penile procedures under local anesthesia	**Technique(s)**
Circumcision	Penile block and local infiltration
Meatotomy	Spongiosal block and local infiltration
Prosthesis insertion	Crural block and local infiltration
Dorsal slit	Penile block and local infiltration
Penile vascular procedures	Penile block and local infiltration

Table 2. Some of the common penile procedures performed under local anesthesia and technique of anesthesia

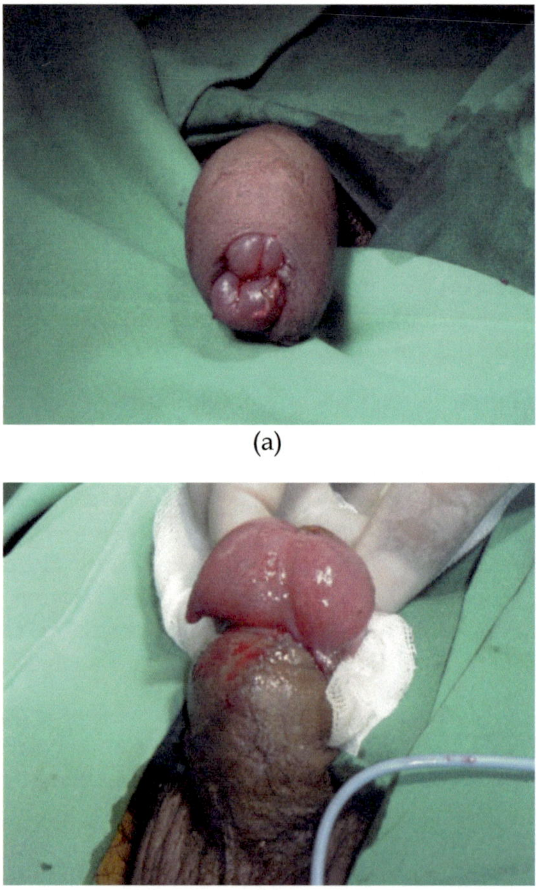

(a)

(b)

Fig. 1. A young man presented in emergency with paraphimosis (a) and had Dorsal slit surgery (b) under local anesthesia

Local anesthesia for penile implants has been substantially reported; its methodology, simplicity and reliability left room for improvement. Hsu and colleagues (Hsu et al., 2004) reported an innovative penile crural block using local anesthesia in patients who underwent penile implantation as outpatient surgery. In 21 men with erectile dysfunction surgery was performed under pudendal nerve block as an outpatient procedure. A proximal dorsal nerve block with peripenile infiltration and penile crural block was developed to replace the anesthesia method of pudendal nerve blocks in 137 consecutive patients (aged from 35 to 83 years) undergoing penile implants. The anesthetic effects and postoperative results with the crural block were very satisfactory. Common immediate side effects included puncture of the vessels, subcutaneous ecchymosis, transient palpitations and dilation pain, but there were no significant late complications. This new anesthetic method proved to be reliable, simple, and safe with fewer complications. It offers the advantages of less morbidity, preservation of patient's privacy, reduced adverse effects of anesthesia, and a more-rapid return to activity with minimal complications. Hsu and colleagues (Hsu et al., 2003) performed 29 men with penile deformity, venous patch for morphologic correction. They received autologous grafting of the deep dorsal vein under local anesthesia as an outpatient procedure. The anesthetic effect and postoperative results were satisfactory. The common immediate side effects included puncture of the vessels, subcutaneous ecchymosis, and transient palpitation, but there were no significant late complications. All patients returned home uneventfully. This has been proven to be a cost-effective, simple, and safe method with fewer complications. It offers the advantages of lower morbidity, fewer adverse effects of anesthesia, and a more rapid return to activity with minimal complications.

4. Endoscopic per urethral procedures (table 3)

Endoscopic perurethral procedures	**Technique(s)**
Cystoscopy	Surface anesthesia
Urethrotomy	Surface anesthesia + Spongiosal block
Ureteroscopic stone fragmentation	Sedoanalgesia and surface anesthetic
Cystolitholapexy	Sedoanalgesia and surface anesthetic
Prostate surgery for BPH	Peri prostatic block(10cc 1%lidocaine at the prostatic apex) and surface anesthesia (perianal-intrarectal lidocaine-prilocaine cream) ± sedoanalgesia

Table 3. Endourological procedures under local anesthesia and technique of anesthesia

4.1 Cystoscopy

Cystoscopy is performed both as a diagnostic and therapeutic maneuver. It is frequently used as a surveillance tool for patients with non-muscle invasive bladder cancer. The conventional radiological imaging techniques lack in detection of small lesions in the urinary bladder. In cystoscopy, the urinary bladder is evaluated through urethra with the help of a telescope or microscope attached to the tip of cystoscope, with local anesthesia administered for it most of the times. It is indicated for investigations in cases of urinary tract infections, hematuria, and incontinence, pain during urination, prostate hypertrophy, and calculus in the urinary tract, among others.

Flexible cystoscopy under local anesthesia has been favored against rigid cystoscopy under general anesthesia. On comparing the two with regards to the patient preference, morbidity and post-operative symptoms, the flexible cystoscopy proved to be better (Denholm et al., 1990).

Cystoscopy is chiefly risk-free but may result in urinary tract infection post-procedure (Clark and Higgs, 1990). The procedure is well tolerated and we recently showed that patients if allowed to view the video monitor of the procedure report lower pain on the visual analogue scale (Soomro et al., 2011).

4.1.1 Diagnostic uses

Ranking 4th in the list of most common cancers, bladder cancer has the tendency to recur. The fact given, it is imperative to make maximum efforts to early diagnose the cancer and to not miss out any case during examination. Detection of bladder cancers by different techniques of cystoscopy has been the focus of research for a long time. On comparing hexaminolevulinate (HAL) fluorescence cystoscopy with standard cystoscopy, the former proved to be significantly better for detection of bladder tumors particularly, carcinoma in situ since HAL fluorescence cystoscopy poses no additional complications, it has also been recommended to be an adjunct procedure with standard cystoscopy (Schmidbauer et al., 2004; Jichlinski et al., 2003). In phase III trial, there was one case of bladder cancer that was detected by HAL fluorescence cystoscopy that was missed by white light cystoscopy (Grossman et al., 2007). Study on efficacy of virtual cystoscopy in patients with bladder tumors shows that its use is still in its infancy and has not yet reached the acceptable quality of fibreoptic examination (Merkle et al., 1998). Yet another study found that in comparison with standard cystoscopy, narrow-band imaging could better detect "non-muscle-invasive bladder tumors" (Herr and Donat, 2008). Cystoscopy has specially been advocated for patients with spinal spinal cord injuries with either chronic or recurrent urinary tract infection to check for squamous cell cancer of the urinary bladder (Navon et al., 1997).

4.1.1.1 Hematuria

Cystoscopy as initial diagnostic modality in subjects with asymptomatic microscopic hematuria has its merits even in outpatient clinics despite increased cost of the procedure (Hong et al., 2001), though concerns have been raised on its invasiveness. Work-up on patients with hematuria revealed that virtual cystoscopy is comparable to conventional cystoscopy to detect masses (Fenlon et al., 1997). The most common cause of microscopic hematuria is a tumor in the urinary tract.

4.1.2 Anesthesia during cystoscopy

Due to patient discomfort experienced under local anesthesia during cystoscopy, there at times is a need to resort to general anesthesia. There have been efforts underway to make the procedure more patient-friendly. Choong and associates demonstrated that anesthesia with 20mL of 2% lignocaine gel is more effective when left on for a longer period of time than current practices (Choong et al., 1997). It has been demonstrated that if lignocaine is applied slowly to administer local anesthesia, the patient discomfort lessens (Khan et al., 2002). In a comparison of 2% lignocaine gel with plain lubricating gel during cystoscopy, there was no analgesic difference noted between the two (Birch et al., 1994). It has been suggested that chemical content in lignocaine is the cause of pain during delivery in cystoscopy (Ho et al., 2003). One significant finding in this regard is that if the gel is refrigerated to 4°C, it reduces the discomfort caused by instillation of Lidocaine gel into male urethra (Goel and Aron, 2003).

4.2 Urethrotomy

A study compared the efficacy of optical internal urethrotomy and dilatation for treating urethral strictures, both being carried out under local anesthesia (Steenkamp et al., 1997). In the light of this publication, both procedures fared equally well, reflecting onto the success of local anesthesia. During internal urethrotomy, the complications and failures are more frequent for men that have longer or multiple strictures and those that have positive urine culture. Patients with traumatic strictures and those that haven't undergone any treatment for strictures previously also resulted in lesser success in the same study.

Recently, optical urethrotomy was shown to be a feasible choice with 91% success even in patients with severe urethral strictures. This procedure under local anesthesia was very well tolerated with extremely low complication rate (Munks et al., 2010). Comparatively lesser success was shown in 1993 with topical lidocaine anesthesia that gave a success of 83% (Kreder et al., 1993).

Non-randomized trial on safety and efficacy of optical urethrotomy using local anesthesia, spongiosum block with sedation, (figure 2) for anterior urethral stricture demonstrated that compared to major regional or general anesthesia, this method was equally effective and safe (Ather et al., 2009). Merits of local anesthesia could be shorter operating time and cost-effectiveness (Ather et al., 2009). A new local anesthetic technique of intracorpus spongiosum anesthesia was tested on subjects with anterior urethral stricture and showed promising outcomes with 95.7% patients showing no signs of pain during the procedure and only one case experienced very mild and tolerable pain (Ye and Rong-gui et al., 2002). Analgesia lasted for 1.5 hours by intracorpus spongiosum as opposed to 1 hour in spongiosum block with sedation.

Optical internal urethrotomy was successful in 92.9% cases with short stricture length reported in 2007. This minimally invasive procedure was suggested to be safe and comfortable and yet, inexpensive (Altinova and Turkan, 2007).

A new tool of using the diode laser to treat urethral strictures has been proposed, which was tolerated by only 3 out of 22 patients under local anesthesia. The rest were operated on under general or spinal anesthesia (Kamal, 2001). The procedure has been advocated as a first line treatment.

Another method of local anesthesia, the transperineal urethrosphincteric block using 1% lidocaine showed favorable results in treating anterior urethral strictures, with 92% patients very satisfied with the procedure. No post-operative complications were noted and there was absolutely no need of additional analgesia during the procedure (Al-Hunayan et al., 2008).

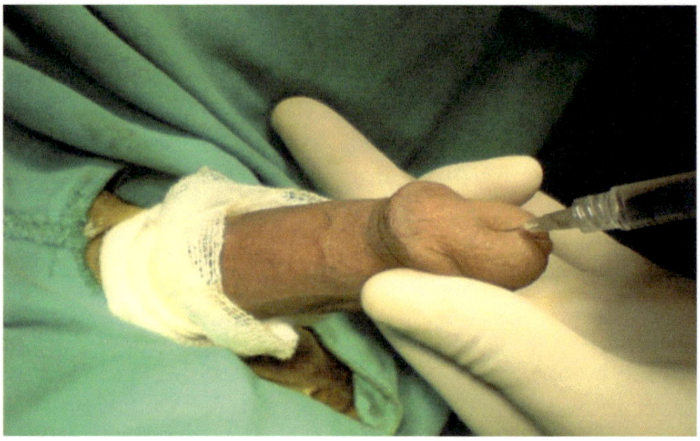

Fig. 2. Spongiosum block being administered using 1% lidocaine without epinephrine in the corpus spongiosum

Urethrotomy should be used only for selected cases to have ideal success rate. Otherwise, an overall low success rate of ±60% has been reported. Only minor complications occur during or following internal urethrotomy, like infections and hemorrhage. The procedure also has other advantages like ease, simplicity and high speed (Naude and Heyns, 2005). Urethroplasty has a higher success rate than urethrotomy, but is not a cost-effective procedure.

Urethral strictures very often recur, and stricture in penile urethra of greater length being a significant risk for recurrence (Zehri et al., 2009). Patients with these risks should undergo alternative procedures.

The reported success of the procedure varies from 66% to 90%. In case of recurrence that occurs very commonly, repeat direct vision internal urethrotomy is of no value at all. But since the procedure is easy, simple and can be done in outpatient setting under local anesthesia, there's evidence that the procedure is being used excessively and inappropriately. Successful management in cases of obliterative strictures less than 1 cm has been demonstrated using flexible cystoscopy guided- internal urethrotomy (Hosseini et al., 2008).

4.2.1 Complications

Common complications following the procedure are: recurrence of stricture which at times, can be worse than the previous one; pain if the procedure is under local anesthesia or pain post-operatively; infections; periurethral abscess; urethral fistula; and bleeding

4.2.2 Success

Despite all its popularity, concerns have been raised recently on its poor performance. The first or any of the repeated urethrotomies didn't have a success that exceeded 9% (Santucci and Eisenberg, 2010). There was one randomized trial testing the efficacy of Mitomycin C application in internal urethrotomy, which showed its success in reducing the rate of recurrence of strictures (Mazdak, 2007).

4.3 Ureteroscopic stone fragmentation

The ureter receives a rich autonomic nerve supply. Unmyelinated nerve fibers are located in the lamina propria, muscle coat, and adventitia of the ureter. The ureter receives preganglionic sympathetic input from the T10 through L2 spinal segments. Postganglionic fibers arise from several ganglia in the celiac, aorticorenal, mesenteric, superior, and inferior hypogastric (pelvic) autonomic plexuses. The upper ureter receives parasympathetic input from vagal fibers by means of the celiac plexus and the lower ureter from the S2 through S4 spinal segments. Afferent nerves from the upper portion of the ureter reach the spinal cord with the sympathetic fibers from the T10 through L2 spinal segments. Afferents from the lower ureter travel by way of the pelvic plexus to the S2 through S4 spinal segments.

Ureterorenoscopy (URS) is an important tool in the diagnosis and management of most uretero renal pathologies. URS with local anesthesia (LA) and intravenous (IV) sedation can be performed as a diagnostic procedure or to manage ureteral and renal calculi, ureteropelvic junction (UPJ) obstruction, ureteral strictures, and small upper tract transitional cell carcinoma (TCC) recurrences. With advances in ureteroscopic design and the introduction of short-acting anesthetics, URS can now be performed efficiently with high patient satisfaction and minimal post operative recovery time. Recently, URS under local anesthesia, with or without sedation, has become a viable option for a high percentage of correctly selected patients.

For URS in selected patients only anesthesia used is surface anesthesia for the urethra. This may be complemented with IV sedation and analgesia. Use of Midazolam has an added advantage that most patients even with fair pain control have modest recollection of the events. Patient selection is vital to a successful procedure. Women with shorter urethra are preferred over men. Distal ureteral stone rather than proximal ureteral stone should be performed under LA. Balloon dilatation is well tolerated but preference should be to use smaller diameter ureteroscopes (≤7.5 Fr).

4.4 Cystolithotripsy

Bladder stones in modern urologic practice are often smaller stones from the upper urinary tract. Larger stones are mostly primary bladder stones as a consequence of neglected bladder outlet obstruction secondary to BPH or neurogenic bladder. Kara and colleagues (Kara et al., 2009) treated 13 patients with transurethral holmium laser cystolithotripsy (HLC) with a flexible cystoscope under local anesthesia. All patients were rendered stone free, regardless of stone size. The mean stone size was 3.6 cm (range 3-5) and the mean operative time was 51 minutes (range 45-65). The whole procedure was well tolerated and no significant differences were found in the mean pain score between the HLC group and a group of male patients that underwent flexible cystoscopy under local anesthesia (2.15

versus 1.86, respectively; p =0.467). No major intraoperative complication occurred. Results of percutaneous approach to bladder stone have similarly been reported with good tolerability and high stone free rate (Tzortzis et al 2006).

4.5 Prostate surgery for BPH

Bladder outlet obstruction secondary to benign prostatic hyperplasia is one of the commonest disorders of the ageing men. Medical management with alpha-blocker s and 5 alpha reductase inhibitors has become the first line in majority of the patients; still significant numbers do require surgical intervention. Open prostatectomy and TURP are considered the gold standard, however, newer less invasive modalities like various forms of laser prostatectomy, trans urethral needle ablation, micro wave thermotherapy, focused ultrasound treatment, ethanol ablation, etc. have been introduced in recent years. Although TURP provides durable results, it is associated with considerable morbidity (Hong et al., 2011). This is of particular concern as most patients needing TURP are old and have multiple co-morbidities.

One of the major advantages of some of these minimally invasive procedures is the ability to perform them under local anesthesia. Transurethral ethanol ablation of the prostate (TEAP) has been introduced as a minimally invasive alternative treatment for patients with BPH. El-Husseiny and Buchholz (El-Husseiny and Buchholz, 2011) used dehydrated ethanol in a concentration of 95% to 98%, which was injected transurethrally by means of the Postaject Ethanol Injection System using a rigid cystoscope. They reported that there was sufficient response in 73% of their patients, while the remaining 27% showed an insufficient response and needed alternative treatment. Microwave thermotherapy is another minimally invasive therapy for BPH. It can either be performed perurethrally (TUMT) or transperineally. Bartolleti and colleagues (Bartolleti et al., 2008) evaluated the tolerability and safety of a newly designed probe for trans-perineal microwave thermoablation (TPMT) of the prostate in patients with BPH, and the in vivo microwave effects on prostatic tissue using local anesthesia. They reported that no adverse events from TPMT treatment were noted. In particular, no patients reported local, pelvic, or abdominal pain during the procedure or subsequent alterations of defecation rhythm, ano-rectal/intestinal problems, or hematuria. No differences in quality of life or in sexual function were reported. Use of radiofrequency for the treatment of BPH has evolved considerably in the recent years with introduction of newer generation of transurethral needle ablation (TUNA) devices. In the reported work by Zlotta and colleagues (Zlotta et al., 2003) patients were treated using the TUNA II or TUNA III catheters under local anesthesia only without general or spinal anesthesia. The authors reported that TUNA is effective and provides good long-term clinical improvement at 5-year follow-up. TUNA treatment stands the test of time at 5-year follow-up with low and acceptable failure rates. More than 75% of the patients do not need additional treatment for BPH on the long run.

5. Interventional stone treatment

5.1 Extracorporeal shock wave lithotripsy

It was the struggle with urinary tract stones that shaped urology as a separate medical specialty. With the advancement in technology, the role of open surgery has decreased considerably over decades with minimally invasive techniques now the treatment of choice for surgeons (Ather et al., 2001). The minimally invasive procedure of extracorporeal shock-wave lithotripsy (ESWL) was introduced in 1980s and since then, has revolutionized the management of urolithiasis providing virtually ideal outcomes. After extensive trials in vivo and on animal models, its first human trial was carried out in 1980 and its success led to more hope for management of urolithiasis. It is the most commonly undertaken procedure to treat renal stones with a 90% success rate (Ather et al., 2004).

5.1.1 Anesthetic techniques

The entry of shockwaves into the body through water is the most painful part of the procedure, necessitating analgesia. If the power of lithotripter is reduced, the procedure can be conducted without anesthesia but it results in a higher incidence of re-treatments (D'Addessi et al., 2008). For that reason, ESWL is carried out under general anesthesia, epidural anesthesia and spinal anesthesia (Rickford et al., 1988). Initially the procedure was mainly carried out under general anesthesia but with improvement in technology, reports of ESWL with local anesthesia were shown (Madbouly et al., 2011). General anesthesia though faster and more reliable results in more post-operative complications like nausea, vomiting and sore throat (Rickford et al., 1988). A downside of spinal anaethesia is that a significant proportion of patients suffer from postspinal headache (Rickford et al., 1988). Regional and local anesthesia has obvious advantages of having a conscious patient that can assist in the procedure (Rickford et al., 1988). Hypotension during placement in hoist is observed with both general and regional anesthesia (Rickford et al., 1988). A very recent randomized trial tested the efficacy of sub-cutaneous local versus intramuscular opioid sedation and found that the former alone was effective (Madbouly et al., 2011). A eutectic mixture of local anesthetics has been suggested to induce analgesia during ESWL, with clinical use in cases where intravenous analgesia is contraindicated (Bierkens et al., 1991; Keller and Elliot, 1994). Successful experience with local anesthesia for lithotripsy has been reported multiple times (Loening et al., 1987; Keller and Elliot, 1994).

Local anesthesia in carefully selected patients' works well for stones that are moderate size and are not too hard in consistency (Aeikens et al., 1986). Investigators have made the comparison between different techniques for local anesthesia. One such comparison was made between eutectic mixture of local anesthetics and dimethyl sulfoxide with lidocaine (lignocaine), with the latter significantly proven to be better (Demir et al., 2007; Kumar et al., 2010). On the other hand, there have been reports showing that local anesthesia does not decrease the requirement of intravenous analgesia in patients with renal and ureteral stones when using second-generation lithotripter (Turker and Ozgen et al., 2000).

5.2 Percutaneous nephrostolithotomy

Larger renal stone (> 20mm) and those in the lower pole calyx even of 15mm size are preferentially now treated by percutaneous nephrostolithotomy (PCNL). PCNL is typically performed in prone position under general anesthesia. Anesthesia during PCNL for staghorn and large renal stones is a challenge because of the possibility of fluid absorption (Rozentsveig et al., 2007) dilutional anemia, hypothermia, or significant blood loss. There have been few series of PCNL under spinal anesthesia (Mahrabi et al., 2010). In a series of 160 consecutive patients the authors have reported that PCNL under spinal anesthesia is safe and effective for performing PCNL and is a good alternative for general anesthesia in adult patients (Mahrabi et al., 2010). The other complicating factor particularly in obese patients is tube displacement, nerve compression, etc during prone positioning following intubation. Wu and colleagues (Wu et al., 2009) described a technique of awake intubation and prone patient self-positioning before PCNL. They reported that the technique of awake intubation with prone patient self-positioning can be helpful for positioning morbidly obese patients before PCNL and has been safe and effective in properly selected patients. Obesity or prone positioning should not impact efficacy of PCNL and morbidity minimized provided that surgical and anesthesia teams understand and safeguard against potential complications (Wu et al., 2009). In another interesting work Aravantinos and colleagues (Aravantinos et al., 2009) used multimodal anesthesia in order to avoid complications related to general anesthesia. The multimodal analgesic regime used included paracetamol, a COX (2) inhibitor, epidural morphine, and infiltration of the surgical field with local anesthetics (Aravantinos et al., 2009). The use of our multimodal analgesia regime is a well-tolerated and safe alternative to general or regional anesthesia for patients undergoing PCNL.

Aravantinos and colleagues (Aravantinos et al, 2007) performed PCNL under local anesthesia in twenty-four patients with unilateral renal obstruction due to pelvic stones ≥ 2.0 cm. A 16 Ch percutaneous nephrostomy was placed to decompress the obstructed kidney under local anesthesia for 1 week prior to definitive procedure. The tract and the renal parenchyma was infiltrated with lignocaine, dilatation of the nephrostomy tract was performed. Subsequently, PCNL was done using a 24-Fr rigid nephroscope and a ballistic lithotripter. All patients were pre medicated with pethidine HCl intramuscularly 30 min before the beginning of both stages. Diazepam was given (0.1mg/kg orally) to patients before the second stage. Pain scores were collected using 10-cm linear visual analogue scale (VAS) after the completion of both procedures. They noted that the mean VAS score was 38 mm (range: 17-60 mm) for the first stage and 36 mm (13-69 mm) for the second stage. The mean operative time, including both stages, was 127 min (85-155 min). Authors reported no anesthesia-related complications. In another interesting work (Chen et al., 2011) described the feasibility of minimally invasive PCNL under peritubal anesthesia. They performed ureteral catheterization under 1% Lidocaine surface analgesia with pethidine pre medication. The tract was infiltrated with 1% Lidocaine using spinal needle from renal parenchyma, capsule to skin surface. The authors reported that the procedure is well-tolerated and feasible alternative to general and epidural anesthesia.

6. Conclusion

The impetus for urological procedures under local anesthesia has been to maximize anesthetic and postoperative resources by increasing patient turnover in the operating room and discharging patients' home more efficiently on the same day. This is of particular importance due to increasing burden on the health care structure. In addition, patients with significant co morbidities, with relative or absolute contra indication to general or major regional anesthesia can also undergo procedures safely. The use of local anesthesia has continued to expand the ability of urologists to perform a variety of procedures in a safer fashion, particularly in high-risk patients. Additional advantages of local anesthesia include the avoidance of postoperative nausea and vomiting with early resumption of a normal diet, an enhanced ability to perform the surgical procedure on an outpatient basis with early discharge, a lower risk of intra operative complications (cardiac and pulmonary), the ability to communicate with the patient during the procedure, and an enhanced perception that the procedure will not be associated with a prolonged postoperative recovery period.

7. References

Aeikens, B., Fritz, KW. & Hoehne, E. (1986). Initial experience with local anesthesia in extracorporeal shock wave lithotripsy, *Urol Int.* Vol.41(No. 4): 246-7

Al-Hunayan, A., Al-Awadi, K., Al-Khayyat, A. & Abdulhalim, H. (2008). A pilot study of transperineal urethrosphincteric block for visual internal urethrotomy in patients with anterior urethral strictures, J Endourol Vol.22(No.5): 1017-20.

Altinova, S. & Turkan, S. (2007). Optical urethrotomy using topical anesthesia, Int Urol Nephrol Vol.39(No.2): 511-2.

Amory, JK., Jessen, JW., Muller, C. & Berger, RE. (2010). Vasectomy by epithelial curettage without suture or cautery: a pilot study in humans, Asian J Androl Vol.12(No. 3): 315-21

Aravantinos, E., Kalogeras, N., Stamatiou, G., Theodorou, E., Moutzouris, G., Karatzas, A. & Melekos, M. (2009). Percutaneous nephrolithotomy under a multimodal analgesia regime, *J Endourol* Vol.23(No. 5): 853-6.

Aravantinos E, Karatzas A, Gravas S, Tzortzis V. & Melekos M. (2007) Feasibility of percutaneous nephrolithotomy under assisted local anaesthesia: a prospective study on selected patients with upper urinary tract obstruction. *Eur Urol.* Vol. 51, (No.1):pp.224-7

Ather, MH., Faruqui, N., Akhtar, S. & Sulaiman, MN. (2004). Is an excretory urogram mandatory in patients with small to medium-sized renal and ureteric stones treated by extra corporeal shock wave lithotripsy? *BMC Med Vol.*28(No. 2):15.

Ather, MH., Paryani, J., Memon, A. & Sulaiman, MN. (2001). A 10-year experience of managing ureteric calculi: changing trends towards endourological intervention--is there a role for open surgery? *BJU Int* Vol.88(No. 3): 173-7

Ather, MH., Zehri, AA., Soomro, K. & Nazir, I. (2009). The safety and efficacy of optical urethrotomy using a spongiosum block with sedation: a comparative nonrandomized study, *J Urol* Vol.181(No. 5): 2134-8.

Bartoletti, R., Cai, T., Tinacci, G., Longo, I., Ricci, A., Massaro, MP., Tosoratti, N., Zini, E. & Pinzi, N. (2008). Transperineal microwave thermoablation in patients with obstructive benign prostatic hyperplasia: a phase I clinical study with a new mini-choked microwave applicator, *J Endourol* Vol.22(No. 7): 1509-17.

Beiko, DT., Kim, D. & Morales, A. (2003). Aspiration and sclerotherapy versus hydrocelectomy for treatment of hydroceles, *Urology* Vol.61(No. 4): 708-12.

Bierkens, AF., Maes, RM., Hendrikx, JM., Erdos, AF., de Vries, JD. & Debruyne, FM. (1991). The use of local anesthesia in second generation extracorporeal shock wave lithotripsy: eutectic mixture of local anesthetics, *J Urol Vol.146*(No. 2): 287-9.

Birch, BR., Ratan, P., Morley, R., Cumming, J., Smart, CJ. & Jenkins, JD. (1994). Flexible cystoscopy in men: is topical anaesthesia with lignocaine gel worthwhile? *Br J Urol* Vol.73(No. 2): 155-9.

Burden, RJ., O'Kelly, SW., Sutton, D. & Cumming, J. (1997). Spermatic-cord block improves analgesia for day-case testicular surgery, *Br J Urol* Vol.80(No. 3):472-5.

Cayan, S., Shavakhabov, S. & Kadioğlu, A. (2009). Treatment of palpable varicocele in infertile men: a meta-analysis to define the best technique, *J Androl* Vol.30(No. 1): 33-40.

Chen, Y., Zhou, Z., Sun, W., Zhao, T. & Wang, H. (2011). Minimally invasive percutaneous nephrolithotomy under peritubal local infiltration anesthesia, *World J Urol* DOI 10.1007/s00345-0011-0730-z

Choong, S., Whitfield, HN., Meganathan, V., Nathan, MS., Razack, A. & Gleeson, M. (1997). A prospective, randomized, double-blind study comparing lignocaine gel and plain lubricating gel in relieving pain during flexible cystoscopy, *Br J Urol* Vol.80(No. 1): 69-71.

Clark, KR. & Higgs, MJ. (1990). Urinary infection following out-patient flexible cystoscopy, *Br J Urol* Vol.66(No. 5): 503-5.

D'Addessi, A., Bongiovanni, L., Sasso, F., Gulino, G., Falabella, R. & Bassi, P. (2008). Extracorporeal shockwave lithotripsy in pediatrics, *J Endourol* Vol.22(No. 1): 1-12.

Demir, E., Kilciler, M., Bedir, S., Erten, K. & Ozgok, Y. (2007). Comparing two local anesthesia techniques for extracorporeal shock wave lithotripsy, *Urology* Vol.69(No. 4): 625-8.

Denholm, SW., Conn, IG., Newsam, JE. & Chisholm, GD. (1990). Morbidity Following Cystoscopy: Comparison of Flexible and Rigid Techniques, *Br J Urol* Vol.66(No. 2): 152-4

Desmond, AD., Arnold, AJ. & Hastie, KJ. (1998). Subcapsular orchiectomy under local anesthesia. Technique, results and implications, *Br J Urol* Vol.61(No. 2): 143-5.

El Hussainey, T. & Buchholz, N. (2011). Transurethral ethanol ablation of the prostate for symptomatic benign prostatic hyperplasia: long-term follow-up, *J Endourol* Vol.25(No. 3): 477-80

Fahmy, I., Kamal, A., Aboulghar, M., Mansour, R., Serour, GI. & Shamloul, R. (2004). Percutaneous aspiration biopsy using an intravenous catheter for testicular sperm retrieval in patients with obstructive azoospermia, *Reprod Biomed Online* Vol.9(No. 1): 102-5.

Fenlon, HM., Bell, TV., Ahari, HK. & Hussain, S. (1997). Virtual cystoscopy: early clinical experience, *Radiology* Vol.205(No. 1): 272-5..

Goel, R. & Aron, M. (2003). Cooled lignocaine gel: does it reduce urethral discomfort during instillation? *Int Urol Nephrol* Vol.35(No. 3): 375-7.

Grossman, HB. (2007). Improving the management of bladder cancer with fluorescence cystoscopy, *J Environ Pathol Toxicol Oncol* Vol.26(No. 2): 143-7.

Herr, HW. & Donat, SM. (2008). A comparison of white-light cystoscopy and narrow-band imaging cystoscopy to detect bladder tumour recurrences, *BJU Int* Vol.102(No. 9): 1111-4.

Ho, KJ., Thompson, TJ., O'Brien, A., Young, MR. & McCleane, G. (2003). Lignocaine gel: does it cause urethral pain rather than prevent it? *Eur Urol* Vol.43(No. 2): 194-6.

Hong, SK., Ahn, C. & Kim, HH. (2001). The value of cystoscopy as an initial diagnostic modality for asymptomatic microscopic hematuria, *J Korean Med Sci* Vol.16(No. 3): 309-12.

Hong, JY., Yang, SC., Ahn, S. & Kil HK. (2011). Preoperative comorbidities and relationship of comorbidities with postoperative complications in patients undergoing transurethral prostate resection, *J Urol* Vol.185(No. 4): 1374-8.

Hosseini, SJ., Kaviani, A. & Vazirnia, AR. (2008). Internal urethrotomy combined with antegrade flexible cystoscopy for management of obliterative urethral stricture, *Urol J* Vol.5(No. 3): 184-7.

Hsu, GL., Hsieh, CH., Wen, HS., Chen, SC., Chen, YC., Liu, LJ., Mok, MS. & Wu, CH. (2004). Outpatient penile implantation with the patient under a novel method of crural block, *Int J Androl* Vol.27(No. 3): 147-51.

Hsu, GL., Hsieh, CH., Chen, HS., Ling, PY., Wen, HS., Liu, LJ., Chen, CW. & Chua, C. (2007). The advancement of pure local anesthesia for penile surgeries: can an outpatient basis be sustainable? *J Androl* Vol.28(No. 1): 200-5.

Hsu, GL., Hsieh, CH., Wen, HS., Hsieh, JT. & Chiang, HS. (2003). Outpatient surgery for penile venous patch with the patient under local anesthesia *J Androl* Vol.24(No. 1): 35-9.

Hsu, GL., Ling, PY., Hsieh, CH., Wang, CJ., Chen, CW., Wen, HS., Huang, HM., Einhorn, EF. & Tseng GF. (2005). Outpatient varicocelectomy performed under local anesthesia, *Asian J Androl* Vol.7(No. 4): 439-44

Jichlinski, P. (2003). New diagnostic strategies in the detection and staging of bladder cancer, *Curr Opin Urol* Vol.13(No. 5): 351-5.

Kamal, BA. (2001). The use of the diode laser for treating urethral strictures, *BJU Int* Vol.87(No. 9): 831-3.

Kara, C., Resorlu, B., Cicekbilek, I. & Unsal, A. (2009). Transurethral cystolithotripsy with holmium laser under local anesthesia in selected patients, *Urology* Vol.74(No. 5): 1000-3.

Keller, RJ. & Elliott, C. (1994). Eutectic mixture of local anesthetic cream--topical anesthesia for extracorporeal shock wave lithotripsy, *CRNA* Vol.5(No. 4): 136-8.

Khan, MA., Beyzade, B., Tau, W., Virdi, JS. & Potluri, BS. (2002). Effect of the rate of delivery of lignocaine gel on patient discomfort perception prior to performing flexible cystoscopy, *Urol Int* Vol.68(No. 3): 164-7

Khaniya, S., Agrawal, CS., Koirala, R., Regmi, R. & Adhikary, S. Comparison of aspiration-sclerotherapy with hydrocelectomy in the management of hydrocele: a prospective randomized study, *Int J Surg* Vol.7(No. 4): 392-5.

Kiesling, VJ Jr., Schroeder, DE., Pauljev, P. & Hull, J. (1984). Spermatic cord block and manual reduction: primary treatment for spermatic cord torsion, *J Urol* Vol.132(No. 5): 921-3.

Kumar, A., Mohanty, NK., Jain, M., Prakash, S. & Arora, RP. (2010). A prospective randomized comparison between early (<48 hours of onset of colicky pain) versus delayed shockwave lithotripsy for symptomatic upper ureteral calculi: a single center experience. *J Endourol* Vol.24(No. 12): 2059-66.

Kreder, KJ., Stack, R., Thrasher, JB. & Donatucci, CF. (1993). Direct vision internal urethrotomy using topical anesthesia, *Urology* 42(No. 5): 548-50.

Labrecque, M., Dufresne, C., Barone, MA. & St-Hilaire, K. (2004). Vasectomy surgical techniques: a systematic review, *BMC Medicine* Vol.2: 21

Loening, S., Kramolowsky, EV. & Willoughby, B. (1987). Use of local anesthesia for extracorporeal shock wave lithotripsy, *J Urol* Vol.137(No. 4): 626-8.

Madbouly, K., Alshahrani, S., Al-Omair, T., Matrafi, HA. & Mansi, M. (2011). Efficacy of local subcutaneous anesthesia versus intramuscular opioid sedation in extracorporeal shockwave lithotripsy: a randomized study, *J Endourol* Vol.25(No. 5): 845-9.

Magoha, GA. (1998). Local infiltration and spermatic cord block for inguinal, scrotal and testicular surgery, *East Afr Med J* Vol.75 (No. 10): 579-81.

Marchal Escalona, C., Chicharro Molero, JA., Martín Morales, A., Del Rosal Samaniego, JM., Díaz Ramírez, F., Ruiz Domínguez, JL. & Burgos Rodríguez, R. (1993). Local anesthesia in the surgical management of hydrocele and cysts of the spermatic cord, *Actas Urol Esp* Vol.17(No. 1): 68-72.

Mazdak, H., Meshki, I. & Ghassami, F. (2007). Effect of mitomycin C on anterior urethral stricture recurrence after internal urethrotomy, *Eur Urol* Vol.51(No. 4): 1089-92;

Mehrabi, S. & Karimzadeh Shirazi, K. (2010). Results and complications of spinal anesthesia in percutaneous nephrolithotomy, *Urol J* Vol.7(No. 1): 22-5.

Merkle, EM., Wunderlich, A., Aschoff, AJ., Rilinger, N., Görich, J., Bachor, R., Gottfried, HW., Sokiranski, R., Fleiter, TR. & Brambs, HJ. (1998). Virtual cystoscopy based on helical CT scan datasets: perspectives and limitations, *Br J Radiol* Vol.71(No. 843): 262-7.

Munks, DG., Alli, MO. & Goad, EH. (2010). Optical urethrotomy under local anaesthesia is a feasible option in urethral stricture disease, *Trop Doct* Vol.40(No. 1): 31-2.

Navon, JD., Soliman, H., Khonsari, F. & Ahlering, T. (1997). Screening cystoscopy and survival of spinal cord injured patients with squamous cell cancer of the bladder, *J Urol* Vol.157(No. 6): 2109-11.

Naudé, AM. & Heyns, CF. (2005). What is the place of internal urethrotomy in the treatment of urethral stricture disease? *Nat Clin Pract Urol* Vol.2(No. 11): 538-45.

Park, H., Park, M. & Park, T. (1998). Two-year experience with ureteral stones: extracorporeal shockwave lithotripsy v ureteroscopic manipulation, *J Endourol* Vol.12(No. 6): 501-4

Rickford, JK., Speedy, HM., Tytler, JA. & Lim M. (1988). Comparative evaluation of general, epidural and spinal anaesthesia for extracorporeal shockwave lithotripsy, *Ann R Coll Surg Engl* Vol.70(No. 2): 69-73.

Roosen, JU., Klarskov, OP. & Mogensen, P. (2005). Subcapsular versus total orchiectomy in the treatment of advanced prostate cancer: a randomized trial, *Scand J Urol Nephrol* Vol.39(No. 6): 464-7.

Quintero, RA., Johnson, MP., Romero, R., Smith, C., Arias, F., Guevara-Zuloaga, F., Cotton, DB. & Evans, MI. (1995). In-utero percutaneous cystoscopy in the management of fetal lower obstructive uropathy, *Lancet* Vol.346(No. 8974): 537-40.

Quintero, RA., Hume, R., Smith, C., Johnson, MP., Cotton, DB., Romero, R. & Evans, MI. (1995). Percutaneous fetal cystoscopy and endoscopic fulguration of posterior urethral valves, *Am J Obstet Gynecol* Vol.172(No. 1 Pt 1): 206-9.

Rozentsveig, V., Neulander, EZ., Roussabrov, E., Schwartz, A., Lismer, L., Gurevich, B., Klein, Y. & Weksler, N. (2007). Anesthetic considerations during percutaneous nephrolithotomy *J Clin Anesth* Vol.19(No. 5): 351-5.

Santucci, R. & Eisenberg, L. (2010). Urethrotomy has a much lower success rate than previously reported, *J Urol* Vol.183(No. 5): 1859-62.

Schmidbauer, J., Witjes, F., Schmeller, N., Donat, R., Susani, M., Marberger, M. & Hexvix PCB301/01 Study Group. (2004). Improved detection of urothelial carcinoma in situ with hexaminolevulinate fluorescence cystoscopy, *J Urol* Vol.171(No. 1): 135-8

Shih, G., Njoya, M., Lessard, M. & Labrecque, M. (2010). Minimizing pain during vasectomy: the mini-needle anesthetic technique, *J Urol* Vol.183(No. 5): 1959-63.

Sokal, DC. & Labrecque, M. (2009). Effectiveness of vasectomy techniques. *Urol Clin North Am* Vol.36(No. 3): 317-29.

Soomro, KQ., Nasir, AR., Ather, MH. (2011). Impact of patient's self-viewing of flexible cystoscopy on pain using a visual analog scale in a randomized controlled trial, *Urology* Vol. 77(No. 1): 21-3.

Steenkamp, JW., Heyns, CF. & de Kock, ML. (1997). Internal urethrotomy versus dilation as treatment for male urethral strictures: a prospective, randomized comparison, *J Urol* Vol.157(No. 1): 98-101.

Taylor, R., Eyres, R., Chalkiadis, GA. & Austin, S. (2003). Efficacy and safety of caudal injection of levobupivacaine, 0.25%, in children under 2 years of age undergoing inguinal hernia repair, circumcision or orchidopexy, *Paediatr Anaesth* Vol.13(No. 2): 114-21.

Türker, AK. & Ozgen S. (2000). Local anesthesia for extracorporeal shock wave lithotripsy: a double-blind, prospective, randomized study, *Eur Urol* Vol.37(No. 3): 331-3.

Tzortzis, V., Aravantinos, E., Karatzas, A., Mitsogiannis, IC., Moutzouris, G. & Melekos, MD. (2006). Percutaneous suprapubic cystolithotripsy under local anesthesia, *Urology* Vol.68(No. 1): 38-41.

Watanabe, M., Nagai, A., Kusumi, N., Tsuboi, H., Nasu, Y. & Kumon, H. (2005). Minimal invasiveness and effectivity of subinguinal microscopic varicocelectomy: a comparative study with retroperitoneal high and laparoscopic approaches, *Int J Urol* Vol.12(No. 10): 892-8.

Weinberg, GL. (2010). Treatment of local anesthetic systemic toxicity (LAST), *Reg Anesth Pain Med* Vol.35(No. 2): 188-93.

Wolfe, JW. & Butterworth, JF. (2011). Local anesthetic systemic toxicity: update on mechanisms and treatment, *Curr Opin Anaesthesiol* [Epub ahead of print].

Wu, SD., Yilmaz, M., Tamul, PC., Meeks, JJ. & Nadler, RB. (2009). Awake endotracheal intubation and prone patient self-positioning: anesthetic and positioning considerations during percutaneous nephrolithotomy in obese patients, *J Endourol* Vol.23(No. 10): 1599-602.

Ye, G. & Rong-gui, Z. (2002). Optical urethrotomy for anterior urethral stricture under a new local anesthesia: intracorpus spongiosum anesthesia, *Urology* Vol.60(No. 2): 245-7.

Zehri, AA., Ather, MH. & Afshan, Q. (2009). Predictors of recurrence of urethral stricture disease following optical urethrotomy, *Int J Surg* Vol.7(No. 4): 361-4.

Zlotta, AR., Giannakopoulos, X., Maehlum, O., Ostrem, T. & Schulman, CC. (2003). Long-term evaluation of transurethral needle ablation of the prostate (TUNA) for treatment of symptomatic benign prostatic hyperplasia: clinical outcome up to five years from three centers, *Eur Urol* Vol.44(No. 1): 89-93.

5

Local Anesthesia for the Prostate Gland

Allison Glass, Sanoj Punnen and Katsuto Shinohara*
Department of Urology, University of California, San Francisco
USA

1. Introduction

The number of prostate biopsies for detection of prostate cancer has been increasing. Local anesthesia prior to biopsy is crucial to improving pain control throughout the procedure. There are many different methods of administering local anesthesia of the prostate and debate still remains regarding the best site for injection, as well as the ideal type and dosage of anesthetic to use for maximum pain relief. Below we outline the history behind local anesthesia of the prostate, the different methods used to administer it and the pros and cons of these approaches.

Prostate cancer is the most common cancer among men in the United States. In 2010 it was estimated that 217, 730 men in the United States were diagnosed with prostate cancer.[1] Although serum prostate specific antigen (PSA) testing and digital rectal exams (DRE) help identify men at risk for prostate cancer the gold standard for diagnosis is currently biopsy of the prostate. With recent trends towards PSA screening there has been an increase in the number of men being diagnosed with prostate cancer and the number of men undergoing biopsy of the prostate. It has been estimated that as many as 800,000 biopsies of the prostate are performed in the United States each year making it one of the most common office procedures for urologists.[2]

Since the majority of prostate cancer foci are not visible on ultrasonography, Hodge et al. proposed systematic sextant random biopsy in order to improve cancer detection rate in 1989.[3] Over the years, the development of prostate biopsy has moved from the original 6 core sextant biopsy to more extended protocols, which allow more extensive sampling of the gland. Most contemporary biopsy protocols today attain 12-16 cores with some protocols advocating for 20 plus cores.[4] Furthermore, the development of active surveillance protocols have required men to undergo serial biopsies as frequently as every 6-12 months to detect tumor progression, making prostate biopsy a frequent procedure for men on such surveillance protocols.

Although biopsy of the prostate has been considered a fairly well tolerated procedure, recent studies have suggested that as many as 90% of patients found the procedure painful.[5] A recent study by Irani et al. reported that 6% of patients felt the procedure should be done under general anesthesia and 19% of patients would refuse the procedure without any analgesia.[6] Furthermore, another study found that 16% of biopsies could not be completed

---

* Corresponding Author

due to pain when anesthesia was not used compared to only 2% of procedures that could not be completed when anesthesia was provided. As a result, the American Urological Association, the European Urological Association and the National Comprehensive Cancer Network currently call for the use of analgesia for pain relief during biopsy of the prostate. Despite this, a recent survey suggested that one third of urologists do not provide any anesthesia during the procedure.[7]

Although there is no consensus on the form or technique used for analgesia, most urologists administer local anesthetic to the prostate prior to biopsy. The most common forms of local anesthesia to the prostate currently include peri-prostatic nerve block, intra-rectal local anesthesia and intra-prostatic injection of local anesthetic. In this review we will discuss the development of local anesthesia of the prostate and the various techniques used to administer it.

2. Anatomy of the prostate

The average prostate weighs 20-25 grams in size in young men and is located just beneath the bladder. It is fixed to the pubic bone anteriorly by the puboprostatic ligaments, cradled laterally by the levators and is directly related to the overlying endopelvic fascia. The prostate is composed of 70% glandular and 30% fibromuscular stroma and can be divided into 4 main zones. The transitional zone, which makes up 5-10% of the gland, surrounds the urethra and is responsible for prostate enlargement problems. It accounts for approximately 20% of prostate cancers. The central zone accounts for 25% of the gland, surrounds the ejaculatory ducts, and is responsible for approximately 1-5% of cancers. The anterior fibromuscular zone does not contain any glandular components but rather muscle and connective tissue. Finally the peripheral zone makes up 70% of the gland, covering the posterolateral aspect of the prostate, and accounts for the majority of prostate cancers.[8]

2.1 Vascular and lymphatic supply

The main arterial blood supply to the prostate is through the prostatic artery, which is a branch of the inferior vesical artery. It divides into a urethral artery and a capsular artery. The urethral artery enters the prostatovesical junction posterolaterally and supplies the transition zone, prostatic urethra and the periurethral glands. The capsular artery runs posterolateral to the prostate with the cavernous nerves in the neurovascular bundle. It pierces the gland at right angles and sends several small branches to the anterior capsule. Venous drainage of the prostate is abundant through the periprostatic plexus. Lymphatic drainage of the prostate is primarily to the obturator and internal iliac lymph nodes.[8]

2.2 Innervation of the prostate

The prostate is thought to have both sympathetic and parasympathetic innervation. Sympathetic fibers come from the grey matter of the last 3 thoracic and first 2 lumbar segments of the spinal cord. They traverse the paravertebral sympathetic chain and reach the pelvic plexus via the superior hypogastric plexus.[9] The parasympathetic fibers originate from the intermediolateral cell column of the second, third and fourth sacral spinal nerves. They arise as pelvic splanchnic nerves that join the hypogastric nerve and branches from the sacral sympathetic ganglia to form the pelvic plexus.[9]

The pelvic plexus sits lateral to the rectum and is perforated by several vessels going to and from various pelvic organs. Its midpoint is at the tips of the seminal vesicles.[10] The caudal portion of the pelvic plexus gives rise to the innervation of the prostate and the cavernous nerves.[11] These nerves pass the tips of the seminal vesicles then lie in the lateral endopelvic fascia near its junction with denonvilliers fascia.[12] They join the capsular artery of the prostate and travel along the posterolateral border of the prostate on the surface of the rectum and make up the neurovascular bundle.[13]

With respect to the sensory innervation of the prostate, neuronal cell bodies that give rise to sensory afferent fibers are not well known. Studies in cats have suggested that over 90% of primary afferent neurons are located in the sacral dorsal root ganglion. It is thought that 70% of these primary sensory afferents project axons to reach the prostate via the pelvic nerve, while 30% project axons via the pudendal nerve. The remaining 10% of primary afferent neurons are found in autonomic neurons in the sympathetic chain ganglia, inferior mesenteric ganglia, and ganglia in the pelvic plexus.[14]

3. Sources of pain

During transrectal ultrasound guided biopsy of the prostate, there are often two sources of pain described by the patient. The first is during insertion of the ultrasound probe into the rectum. This is due to mechanical stretching of the anal canal distal to the dentate line, which is full of sensory fibers.[15] The rectal mucosa above the dentate line has a relatively low sensitivity to pain and it is believed that the pain during biopsy is not closely related to needle penetration of the rectal wall. In contrast, the prostate capsule and parenchyma are very sensitive to pain and needle penetration of the capsule can cause pain via nerve stimulation of sensory receptors in the capsule and transmission of pain through the neurovascular bundle.[15]

A recent study randomized 150 men to no anesthesia, 10 ml of 2% lidocaine gel intra-rectally or a peri-prostatic injection of 5 ml of 1% lidocaine solution prior to ultrasound guided biopsy of the prostate.[16] They found that both groups who received anesthesia reported less pain then the group that did not receive anesthesia. The group that received intra-rectal lidocaine gel reported the least pain with ultrasound probe insertion, while the group that received peri-prostatic lidocaine injection reported the least pain with the actual biopsy. This study lends support to the two different sources of pain described during the biopsy procedure. Innovative techniques to anesthetize the prostate during the procedure tend to address both sources of pain to maximize analgesic affect and tolerability of the procedure.

4. History of prostate local anesthesia

4.1 First utilization

Transrectal ultrasound (TRUS) guided prostatic biopsy came of widespread clinical use in the mid-1980s.[17] Prostate local anesthesia was not common practice until 1996 when Nash et al first described the benefit of prostate nerve block during prostate biopsy.[18] Periprostatic block was achieved by single local injection, on each side of the prostate, into the region of the prostatic pedicle at the base of the prostate just lateral to the junction between the prostate and seminal vesicles. The posterolateral area of fat within the notch between the prostate and seminal vesicle is described as the 'Mount Everest sign' as it creates a hyperechoic pyramid, which can allow for localization of anesthetic placement.[19] The technique was later modified by placing two further depot injections on each side of the prostate on the lateral aspect.[14] Subsequent studies have demonstrated successful periprostatic infiltration only at the apex at the 4 and 8 O' clock positions.[20,21]

4.2 Evolution of prostatic analgesia

After successful application of periprostatic nerve block, different forms of analgesia were investigated. In 2000, Issa et al first described application of intrarectal lidocaine gel during TRUS-guided prostate biopsy.[22] This form of local analgesic was found to be simple, safe and effective in providing satisfactory anesthesia during this procedure. Furthermore, this technique was found to be more convenient, better tolerated and less invasive compared to transrectal and transperineal prostate nerve blocks. Subsequent studies have supported the use of intrarectal anesthetic gel for purposes of prostate biopsy.[16,23] Several researches have successfully improved intrarectal lubricating analgesia by adding topical drugs or compounds. [24-27] Nifedipine blocks slow calcium channels and thus potentially allows for analgesia during probe insertion by way of anal-sphincter relaxation.[27] Topical glyceryl trinitrate (GTN) similarly causes smooth muscle relaxation with subsequent decreases in anal sphincter tone. GTN was found to be safe, easy to handle and effective in pain control during prostatic biopsy. [25,26] Dimethyl sulphoxide (DMSO) is known to facilitate movement of drugs across cell membranes. It has been shown to be effective for musculoskeletal pain when applied topically and has a potential to reduce rectal discomfort.[28] Recently, more attention has been given to using a combination of these approached to maximize anesthetic efficiency and pain relief. In 2001, pelvic plexus block during TRUS-guided prostate biopsy was first described. This approach failed to diminish biopsy-associated pain.[29] Alternatively, several studies did demonstrate success with pelvic plexus block under skilled guidance and doppler ultrasound.[30,31] Caudal block has also been utilized as an approach to anesthetize the prostate as it provides perianal analgesia and anal sphincter relaxation. However, mixed results have been published regarding its efficacy.[32,33]

5. Use of prostatic analgesia

5.1 Local

Periprostatic nerve block has become of widespread use and is the most common form of analgesia for prostatic biopsy.[28,34] One or 2 % lidocaine is typically used as it is effective, economical and safe. Lidocaine also has relatively long duration of action but it is unclear what the optimal dose, concentration and location is for maximum pain relief. The most common injection site is the angle between the prostate base and the seminal vesicles bilaterally.[28]

Lidocaine gel is most widely used lubricating agent during prostate biopsy.[28] This form of prostatic analgesia is considered to be safe, easy to handle and inexpensive. Studies have revealed that this type of anesthetic is effective in controlling pain associated with rectal probe insertion and manipulation.[28]

Caudal block and pudendal nerve block require the presence of an anesthetist as knowledge and individualization of the anatomy is required as well as need for patient monitoring after drug administration during hospitalization.[28]

5.2 Systemic

While early strategies for prostatic analgesia during TRUS-guided biopsy typically involved use of local agents, current investigations are evaluating safety and efficacy of combination and systemic therapies. A meta-analysis done by Maccagnano et al found that pain control seems to be superior with systemic analgesic such as tramadol or combination tramadol, especially with non-steroidal antiinflammatory agents.[28] Nitrous oxide, while not widely available in urology outpatient clinics has shown to be an attractive systemic alternative in several studies.[35-37] Sedoanalgesia with agents such as propofol, fentanyl or midazolam should be reserved for when extensive or repeat biopsies are needed.[17,28]

6. Application of prostate anesthesia

Use of local prostatic analgesia has successfully extended beyond TRUS-guided prostatic biopsy alone. Local prostatic analgesia has been proven to provide safe and effective pain relief during other minimally invasive procedures of the prostate, including various procedures used to treat symptomatic benign prostatic hypertrophy (BPH). Historically, these procedures are accomplished by way of general and/or regional systemic analgesia. There is now greater recognition of the potential to use local analgesia because of cost- effectiveness and relatively fewer contraindications to local rather than systemic or regional anesthesia.

Periprostatic nerve block has been shown to be effective during transurethral resection of the prostate (TURP).[38,39] Kedia[40] described a local analgesic protocol that was safe, economical, and an effective way to perform interstitial laser coagulation for treating BPH. Other minimally invasive treatments for BPH have been preformed successfully under local anesthesia with good results including transperineal microwave ablation of the prostate, radiofrequency-induced thermotherapy of the prostate, transurethral ethanol ablation of the prostate, photoselective prostate vaporization and transurethral needle ablation of the prostate.[41-45]

Furthermore, studies have shown that periprostatic nerve block can successfully be applied to procedures such as internal urethrotomy, transurethral incision of prostate and bladder biopsies or fulguration while providing excellent pain relief. Periprostatic nerve block has also been used effectively for other urologic procedures such as the placement of intraprostatic fiducial markers prior to external beam radiotherapy.[46 47] Local anesthesia of the prostate has also been used for brachytherapy and cyroablation of the prostate with a high degree of patient satisfaction and cost-effectiveness.[48,49]

7. Technique

7.1 Peri-prostatic nerve block

The first description of peri-prostatic injection was by Nash et al. who described bilateral injections between the base of the prostate and the seminal vesicles (Figure 1).[18] The original study reported a decrease in pain on the side that was injected with local anesthetic compared to the side that was not. This was modified by Soloway and Obek, who proposed two additional injections on each side, with one at the midgland and one at the apex of the prostate.[14] Peri-prostatic nerve block works by anesthetic blockage of capsular sensory fibers, resulting in less pain, anxiety and more relaxation of the pelvic muscles, making the procedure more tolerable.

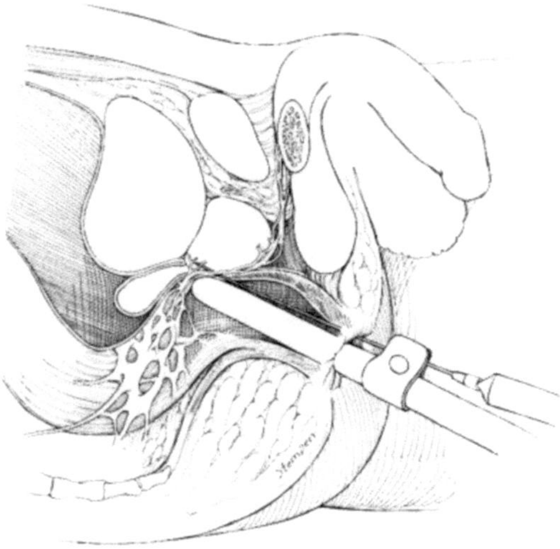

J Urol. Feb 1996;155(2):607-609 with permission

Fig. 1. Ultrasound probe in situ and spinal needle placement within neurovascular bundle at base of prostate just lateral to junction between prostate and seminal vesicle (Reproduced from *Transrectal ultrasound guided prostatic nerve blockade eases systematic needle biopsy of the prostate* by Nash et al.)

Since its first description by Nash et al, multiple studies have tested the efficacy of peri-prostatic nerve block. A recent study randomized 90 patients to no anesthesia, peri-prostatic injection with saline and peri-prostatic injection with 1% lidocaine 5 minutes before biopsy and used a visual analog scale to assess pain.[50] They reported a significant reduction in pain for those men who received peri-prostatic injection of anesthetic. This study has been supported by many meta-analysis, which have showed a benefit in pain reduction during biopsy with peri-prostatic injection of local anesthetic compared to placebo or no anesthesia.[51-53] A recent meta-analysis involving 20 studies and 1685 patients found a significant reduction in pain (weighted mean difference of -2.09, 95% CI -2.44 to -1.75, $p<0.0001$ on a 10 point scale) when comparing peri-prostatic nerve block to no anesthesia or placebo.[53] These authors found similar benefits for peri-prostatic nerve block over no anesthesia or placebo regardless of the site injected.

Studies have also compared the efficacy of peri-prostatic nerve block to intra-rectal anesthetic. Song et al conducted a placebo controlled randomized trial where men were given either 20 ml 2% lidocaine gel intra-rectally, a peri-prostatic injection of 5 ml of 2% lidocaine delivered near the junction of the seminal vesicle and base of the prostate, or a peri-prostatic injection of 5 ml of normal saline injected in a similar location prior to prostate biopsy.[54] They reported a benefit of peri-prostatic nerve block with lidocaine over placebo injection and intra-rectal lidocaine gel. They did not find a benefit for intra-rectal lidocaine gel over placebo injection. These results are supported by a meta-analysis of 6 studies with 872 patients comparing peri-prostatic nerve block to intra-rectal local anesthetic.[53] The authors reported a weighted mean difference of -1.53, 95% CI -2.67 to -0.39 ($p=0.008$), on a 10 point scale in favor of peri-prostatic nerve block over intra-rectal local anesthetic.

Currently there is much variation reported on the ideal location for injection to provide maximum pain relief throughout the biopsy procedure. The initial description by Nash et al suggested bilateral injections between the base of the prostate and seminal vesicles.[18] Since then many studies have advocated for more apical injections.[55,56] The neurovascular bundles run postero-lateral to the prostate gland between the capsule and Denovilllier's fascia and pierce the capsule at the base and apically at the 4 and 8 o'clock location. It has been suggested that injection at these locations will numb the whole gland.[20] A recent study randomized 60 men to bilateral basal injections and 57 men to a single apical injection and found a significant benefit for men who received a single apical injection (p=0.01).[55] The other benefit for a single apical injection was less anesthetic required. This was supported by a study involving 386 men, who were randomized to receive no anesthetic, 10 ml of 1% lidocaine at the apical region of the prostate, 5 ml of 1% lidocaine at the bases of the prostate bilaterally, and lastly 4 ml at the apex and 3 ml at the bases bilaterally of 1% lidocaine.[56] The authors found that 10 ml of apical local anesthetic had the most superior pain relief. However, other studies have not supported this finding. For instance, a study by Philip et al randomized143 men to either apical or basal injections and found no significant difference in pain relief between the two (p=0.36). Currently, the location of injection to induce maximal pain relief is still debatable.

Several studies have assessed the most appropriate dosage of local anesthetic for pain relief during the procedure. Ozden et al randomized 175 men to receive either 2.5 ml, 5 ml or 10 ml of 1% lidocaine and found that 10 ml of local anesthetic provided significantly better pain relief then lower doses.[57] The authors felt that 2.5 ml of local anesthetic was probably not very effective. It has also been suggested that the use of longer acting anesthetics, like bupivacaine, in combination with shorter acting agents can provide longer lasting analgesia and decrease post biopsy discomfort while acting as fast as shorter acting agents.[58] There is still much variation among urologists as to the dose, concentration and type of local anesthetic used.

7.2 Intra-rectal local anesthetic

Another method of providing pain relief during the procedure is to deliver 10-20 ml of intra-rectal gel containing local anesthetic before the procedure. This works to anesthetize the sensory fibers in the anal canal below the dentate line and serves mainly to decrease pain during insertion of the ultrasound probe. Intra-rectal application of lidocaine jelly prior to biopsy was first described by Issa et al, who demonstrated reduced discomfort and pain during the procedure.[22] This was supported by a study involving 80 men who were randomized to either no anesthesia or peri-anal or intra-rectal local anesthetic. The authors reported that peri-anal anesthesia may solely be sufficient to decrease the pain during prostate biopsy. A recent meta-analysis involving 5 studies and 466 patients found the intra-rectal local anesthetic provided better pain relief then no anesthetic or placebo, but the weighted mean difference between the groups did not reach statistical significance.[53] Other studies have suggested that intra-rectal local anesthetic alone is not sufficient for pain relief during the biopsy procedure.[59] Although it works well to reduce the pain associated with probe insertion it does not address the pain associated with injection of the prostate capsule.

7.3 Combination peri-prostatic block and intra-rectal local anesthetic

Contemporary protocols have suggested a combination of peri-prostatic nerve block and intra-rectal local anesthetic prior to biopsy of the prostate. This is thought to provide the most efficient relief of pain during the procedure by addressing the two sources of pain individually (probe insertion and injection into prostate capsule). Obek et al found that the combination of peri-prostatic block and intra-rectal lidocaine worked better then peri-prostatic block alone in a randomized study of 300 men.[60] This is supported by a study involving 223 men showing that peri-prostatic nerve block in addition to intra-rectal local anesthetic provided superior pain relief compared to peri-prostatic nerve block and intra-rectal placebo.[61] Raber et al, noticed a similar benefit to combined peri-prostatic nerve block and intra-rectal local anesthetic over peri-prostatic nerve block alone especially with respect to pain during insertion of the ultrasound report.[62] This lends support to local anesthesia protocols that address both sources of pain during the biopsy procedure. Giannarini et al. reported a randomized study of combination perianal anesthetic cream and periprostatic nerve block. Interestingly in this study, the group with perianal-intrarectal anesthetic cream application had reduced pain score associated with periprostatic block and prostate biopsy. These results suggest that a large dose of lidocaine-prilocaine (5g) intrarectal application 30 minutes prior to the procedure itself can achieve certain anesthetic effect on not only the procto canal but also the prostate gland.[63]

7.4 Intra-prostatic injection of local anesthetic

The first use of intra-prostatic injection was described by Mutaguchi et al. who observed a significant benefit in 71 patients who received intra-prostatic injection from 2002-2003 compared to 99 patients who received traditional peri-prostatic injection from 2001-2002.[64] Intra-prostatic injection provides local anesthetic to sensory fibers within the parenchyma of the prostate, which have a high sensitivity to pain. Secondly, peri-prostatic nerve block does not anesthetize the anterior part of the gland, while intra-prostatic injection does. A randomized, double-blind, 3-arm parallel group study compared 243 men randomized to intra-prostatic injection of local anesthetic, peri-prostatic block to the apical region of the prostate, and peri-prostatic block to the base of the prostate.[65] The authors found that intra-prostatic injection provided superior pain relief compared to basal blockade and similar pain relief to apical blockade.

Other studies have suggested that a combination of intra-prostatic injection and peri-prostatic injection of local anesthetic provides superior pain relief then either alone.[66-68] For example, Binggian et al. randomized 300 men to peri-prostatic and intra-prostatic local anesthetic versus peri-prostatic local anesthetic and intra-prostatic saline.[66] They reported significantly less pain in the group that received combined peri-prostatic and intra-prostatic local anesthetic. Cam et al. found a similar benefit with combined intra-prostatic and peri-prostatic blockade over peri-prostatic blockade alone with no increase in morbidity.[67] Finally, a recent study randomizing 152 patients to either intra-prostatic local anesthetic and peri-prostatic placebo injection, intra-prostatic placebo injection and peri-prostatic local anesthetic or intra-prostatic and peri-prostatic local anesthetic found a significant benefit in pain relief in men who received combined intra-prostatic and peri-prostatic local anesthetic to just peri-prostatic or intra-prostatic local anesthetic alone.[68]

Current Protocol for Local Anesthesia of the Prostate at University of California, San Francisco (UCSF)

Currently, at UCSF, we use a combination of intra-rectal local anesthetic, periprostatic nerve block and intra-prostatic injection of anesthetic to provide fast and efficient relief of pain throughout the procedure (see Figure 2). We use intra-rectal 20% Benzocaine cream applied to the procto canal at the time of the digital rectal examination prior to the ultrasound procedure. Benzocaine is a fast acting mucosal anesthetic achieving effective pain relief in 30 seconds to help minimize pain during probe insertion. Currently, a 1% lidocaine 20 cc solution without sodium bicarbonate or epinephrine is used. About 4cc of the solution is injected in the periprostatic fat at the lateral aspect of prostate and seminal vesicle junction bilaterally (see Figure 3). The rest of the solution is directly injected into the prostate at three locations in each lobe by inserting 22G needle all the way to the anterior capsule at the base, mid gland and the apex, and as the needle is pulled back about 2 cc of anesthetics is slowly infiltrated in the prostate parenchyma at each location. By doing this, systemic circulation of anesthetics can be avoided, and anesthetize the entire gland including the anterior part.

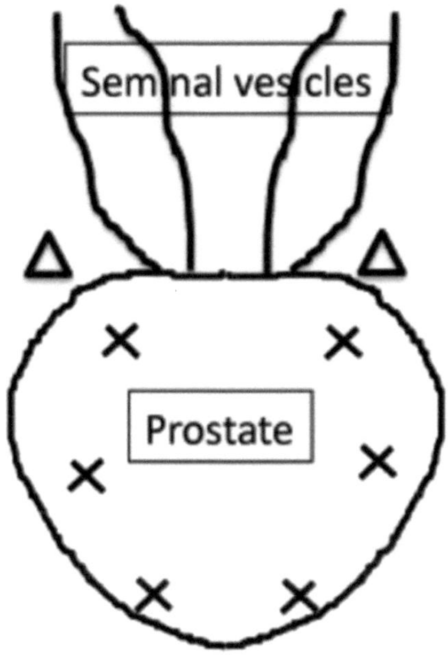

Fig. 2. Local prostatic anesthesia; X's represent intraprostatic injection sites, Triangles represent periprostatic injection sites

8. Complications

There has been comparatively little emphasis placed on evaluation of complications from local prostatic analgesia. Current studies suggest that most forms of local prostatic analgesia are generally safe and well tolerated.[69] The reported complication rate associated with periprostatic nerve block ranges from 2-4%.[17,20,69,70] No significant complication differences were found with intraprostatic analgesia injection[64,67,68] or topical agents.[22,63,71] Of note, reported morbidity is confounded by the fact that many of the complications (i.e. bleeding, infection) can result from the prostatic biopsy itself (i.e. without use of anesthetic).

8.1 Pain

A short-lived, mild "stinging" sensation during injection of the periprostatic nerve block has been reported in the current literature.[20] One study found that about a third of patients undergoing TRUS-guided prostate biopsy experienced discomfort upon injection of analgesic.[69] There are no studies that have documented persistent pain from any form of prostatic analgesia

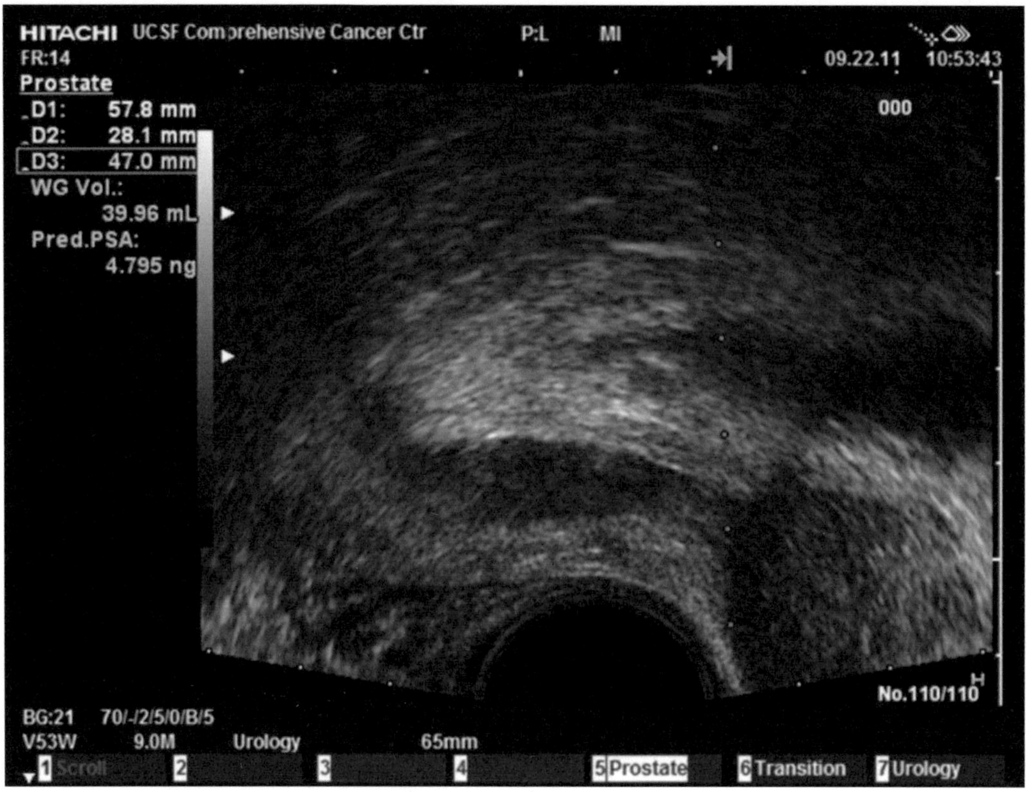

Fig. 3. Ecographic longitudinal image of prostate injection site demonstrating fat plane between prostate and seminal vesicle

8.2 Bleeding

While bleeding can be associated with TRUS-guided prostatic biopsy,[54,72] no reports of significant bleeding attributed to administration of prostatic analgesia have been reported. One study compared complication rates according to number of injections and found no increase in bleeding with greater number of injections.[57] Obek et al actually found a decrease in the incidence of bleeding in patients who received periprostatic nerve block which was explained by improved patient comfort resulting in less movement during the procedure.[70]

8.3 Infection

As the rectum is highly colonized by bacteria, it was questioned whether periprostatic analgesia was associated with high infection rate.[70] The current literature generally disproves this theory.[20,57,73] Conversely, Obek et al did find the incidence of bacteruria, high fever and hospitalization to be higher in the anesthesia group but none of these findings were statistically significant.[70]

8.4 Urinary symptoms

Transient urinary incontinence was reported in 1.5% of patients within first 10 minutes after injection of anesthetic.[69] It was further recommended that patients undergo pre-procedure micturition. Other reports found no change in post biopsy continence after perioprostatic local anesthesia.[74]

8.5 Systemic toxicity

Systemic toxicity results from accidental intravascular injection of anesthetic agent. Clinically, this can appear as dizziness, visual disturbance, tinnitus, metallic taste, lightheadedness, diaphoresis or respiratory distress. The reported incidence of anesthetic toxicity from periprostatic nerve block ranges from 2%-4%.[17,20,70] Vasovagal syncope was reported in as high as 1% of patients,[54] however, vasovagal responses without the application of anesthetic have been reported as well.[69] In addition to aspiration prior to injection, Seymour et al suggested the use of color doppler ultrasound to prevent accidental intravascular injection.[20]

8.6 Other considerations

Authors have expressed concern that minute amounts of air that can potentially be injected during periprostatic analgesia, creating significant image artifacts. Several studies disclaim this. Risk of image artifacts can further be reduced with careful bleeding of the syringe prior to injection and assurance that anesthetic agent is injected outside of the gland.[28] Studies have also reported no difference in intraoperative findings such as fibrosis or loss of planes between the rectum and prostate at radical prostatectomy after prostate biopsy with local anesthetic.[53]

9. Conclusion

With increasing trends towards PSA screening and more utilization of active surveillance protocols for low volume minimal risk disease the number of prostate biopsies being performed are increasing. Contemporary biopsy protocols are calling for more cores and extended sampling of the peripheral zone compared to the previous sextant description. Although once considered a fairly benign procedure, most patients find biopsy of the prostate to be painful and have expressed a desire to be given some anesthetic for pain relief. Most guidelines now consider anesthesia to be a standard of care when performing biopsy of the prostate as it provides better comfort throughout the procedure and less movement of the patient allowing for better visualization of the prostate during the biopsy. Most urologists provide local anesthesia of the prostate of which the most common type is peri-prostatic blockade. There is still some debate as to the best site for injection as well as the type and dosage of local anesthetic to use. Contemporary studies have suggested that combined anesthesia with peri-rectal anesthetic jelly/cream application and peri-prostatic block provides good pain relief by addressing sources of pain from both the rectal probe insertion and the biopsy itself. However, several studies have suggested that any form of local anesthesia is better than no anesthesia and urologists should use whatever method they are comfortable with. To not provide our patients with some form of local anesthetic for pain would be consider beneath most standards of care today.

10. References

[1] Jemal A, Siegel R, Xu J, Ward E. Cancer statistics, 2010. *CA Cancer J Clin.* Sep-Oct 2010;60(5):277-300.

[2] Halpern E, Strup S. Using gray-scale and color and power Doppler sonography to detect prostatic cancer. *AJR Am J Roentgenol.* 2000;174:623-627.

[3] Hodge KK, McNeal JE, Terris MK, Stamey TA. Random systematic versus directed ultrasound guided transrectal core biopsies of the prostate. *J Urol.* Jul 1989;142(1):71-74; discussion 74-75.

[4] Rodriguez-Covarrubias F, Gonzalez-Ramirez A, Aguilar-Davidov B, Castillejos-Molina R, Sotomayor M, Feria-Bernal G. Extended sampling at first biopsy improves cancer detection rate: results of a prospective, randomized trial comparing 12 versus 18-core prostate biopsy. *The Journal of urology.* Jun 2011;185(6):2132-2136.

[5] Clements R, Aideyan OU, Griffiths GJ, Peeling WB. Side effects and patient acceptability of transrectal biopsy of the prostate. *Clin Radiol.* Feb 1993;47(2):125-126.

[6] Collins GN, Lloyd SN, Hehir M, McKelvie GB. Multiple transrectal ultrasound-guided prostatic biopsies--true morbidity and patient acceptance. *Br J Urol.* Apr 1993;71(4):460-463.

[7] Davis M, Sofer M, Kim SS, Soloway MS. The procedure of transrectal ultrasound guided biopsy of the prostate: a survey of patient preparation and biopsy technique. *The Journal of urology.* Feb 2002;167(2 Pt 1):566-570.

[8] Brooks J. *Campbell-Walsh urology / editor-in-chief, Alan J. Wein ; editors, Louis R. Kavoussi ... [et al.].* 9th ed. Philadelphia: W.B. Saunders; 2007.

[9] Benoit G, Merlaud L, Meduri G, et al. Anatomy of the prostatic nerves. *Surg Radiol Anat.* 1994;16(1):23-29.

[10] Schlegel PN, Walsh PC. Neuroanatomical approach to radical cystoprostatectomy with preservation of sexual function. *The Journal of urology.* Dec 1987;138(6):1402-1406.

[11] Walsh PC, Lepor H, Eggleston JC. Radical prostatectomy with preservation of sexual function: anatomical and pathological considerations. *Prostate.* 1983;4(5):473-485.

[12] Lepor H, Gregerman M, Crosby R, Mostofi FK, Walsh PC. Precise localization of the autonomic nerves from the pelvic plexus to the corpora cavernosa: a detailed anatomical study of the adult male pelvis. *The Journal of urology.* Feb 1985;133(2):207-212.

[13] Davies MR. Anatomy of the nerve supply of the rectum, bladder, and internal genitalia in anorectal dysgenesis in the male. *J Pediatr Surg.* Apr 1997;32(4):536-541.

[14] Soloway MS, Obek C. Periprostatic local anesthesia before ultrasound guided prostate biopsy. *J Urol.* Jan 2000;163(1):172-173.

[15] Shinohara K. Pain: easing the pain: local anesthesia for prostate biopsy. *Nat Rev Urol.* Jul 2009;6(7):360-361.

[16] Stirling BN, Shockley KF, Carothers GG, Maatman TJ. Comparison of local anesthesia techniques during transrectal ultrasound-guided biopsies. *Urology.* Jul 2002;60(1):89-92.

[17] Aus G, Damber JE, Hugosson J. Prostate biopsy and anaesthesia: an overview. *Scand J Urol Nephrol.* 2005;39(2):124-129.

[18] Nash PA, Bruce JE, Indudhara R, Shinohara K. Transrectal ultrasound guided prostatic nerve blockade eases systematic needle biopsy of the prostate. *J Urol.* Feb 1996;155(2):607-609.

[19] Jones JS, Oder M, Zippe CD. Saturation prostate biopsy with periprostatic block can be performed in office. *J Urol.* Nov 2002;168(5):2108-2110.
[20] Seymour H, Perry MJ, Lee-Elliot C, Dundas D, Patel U. Pain after transrectal ultrasonography-guided prostate biopsy: the advantages of periprostatic local anaesthesia. *BJU Int.* Oct 2001;88(6):540-544.
[21] Rodriguez A, Kyriakou G, Leray E, Lobel B, Guille F. Prospective study comparing two methods of anaesthesia for prostate biopsies: apex periprostatic nerve block versus intrarectal lidocaine gel: review of the literature. *Eur Urol.* Aug 2003;44(2):195-200.
[22] Issa MM, Bux S, Chun T, et al. A randomized prospective trial of intrarectal lidocaine for pain control during transrectal prostate biopsy: the Emory University experience. *J Urol.* Aug 2000;164(2):397-399.
[23] Mallick S, Humbert M, Braud F, Fofana M, Blanchet P. Local anesthesia before transrectal ultrasound guided prostate biopsy: comparison of 2 methods in a prospective, randomized clinical trial. *J Urol.* Feb 2004;171(2 Pt 1):730-733.
[24] Demir E, Kilicer M, Bedir S, Kilciler G, Erten K, Ozgok Y. Pain scores and local anesthesia for transrectal ultrasound-guided prostate biopsy in patients with anorectal pathologies. *J Endourol.* Nov 2007;21(11):1367-1369.
[25] McCabe JE, Hanchanale VS, Philip J, Javle PM. A randomized controlled trial of topical glyceryl trinitrate before transrectal ultrasonography-guided biopsy of the prostate. *BJU Int.* Sep 2007;100(3):536-538; discussion 538-539.
[26] Brewster S, Rochester M. A randomized controlled trial of topical glyceryl trinitrate before transrectal ultrasonography-guided biopsy of the prostate. *BJU Int.* Dec 2007;100(6):1412-1413.
[27] Cantiello F, Imperatore V, Iannuzzo M, et al. Periprostatic nerve block (PNB) alone vs PNB combined with an anaesthetic-myorelaxant agent cream for prostate biopsy: a prospective, randomized double-arm study. *BJU Int.* May 2009;103(9):1195-1198.
[28] Maccagnano C, Scattoni V, Roscigno M, et al. Anaesthesia in transrectal prostate biopsy: which is the most effective technique? *Urol Int.* 2011;87(1):1-13.
[29] Wu CL, Carter HB, Naqibuddin M, Fleisher LA. Effect of local anesthetics on patient recovery after transrectal biopsy. *Urology.* May 2001;57(5):925-929.
[30] Akpinar H, Tufek I, Atug F, Esen EH, Kural AR. Doppler ultrasonography-guided pelvic plexus block before systematic needle biopsy of the prostate: A prospective randomized study. *Urology.* Aug 2009;74(2):267-271 e261.
[31] Adsan O, Inal G, Ozdogan L, Kaygisiz O, Ugurlu O, Cetinkaya M. Unilateral pudendal nerve blockade for relief of all pain during transrectal ultrasound-guided biopsy of the prostate: a randomized, double-blind, placebo-controlled study. *Urology.* Sep 2004;64(3):528-531.
[32] Horinaga M, Nakashima J, Nakanoma T. Efficacy compared between caudal block and periprostatic local anesthesia for transrectal ultrasound-guided prostate needle biopsy. *Urology.* Aug 2006;68(2):348-351.
[33] Ikuerowo SO, Popoola AA, Olapade-Olaopa EO, et al. Caudal block anesthesia for transrectal prostate biopsy. *Int Urol Nephrol.* Mar 2010;42(1):19-22.
[34] Heidenreich A, Bellmunt J, Bolla M, et al. EAU Guidelines on Prostate Cancer. P5art I: Screening, Diagnosis, and Treatment of Clinically Localised Disease. *Actas Urol Esp.* Jul 12 2011.

[35] Masood J, Shah N, Lane T, Andrews H, Simpson P, Barua JM. Nitrous oxide (Entonox) inhalation and tolerance of transrectal ultrasound guided prostate biopsy: a double-blind randomized controlled study. *J Urol.* Jul 2002;168(1):116-120; discussion 120.
[36] McIntyre IG, Dixon A, Pantelides ML. Entonox analgesia for prostatic biopsy. *Prostate Cancer Prostatic Dis.* 2003;6(3):235-238.
[37] Manikandan R, Srirangam SJ, Brown SC, O'Reilly PH, Collins GN. Nitrous oxide vs periprostatic nerve block with 1% lidocaine during transrectal ultrasound guided biopsy of the prostate: a prospective, randomized, controlled trial. *J Urol.* Nov 2003;170(5):1881-1883; discussion 1883.
[38] Sinha B, Haikel G, Lange PH, Moon TD, Narayan P. Transurethral resection of the prostate with local anesthesia in 100 patients. *J Urol.* Apr 1986;135(4):719-721.
[39] Gorur S, Inanoglu K, Akkurt BC, Candan Y, Kiper AN. Periprostatic nerve blockage reduces postoperative analgesic consumption and pain scores of patients undergoing transurethral prostate resection. *Urol Int.* 2007;79(4):297-301.
[40] Kedia KR. Local anesthesia during interstitial laser coagulation of the prostate. *Rev Urol.* 2005;7 Suppl 9:S23-28.
[41] Bartoletti R, Cai T, Tinacci G, et al. Transperineal microwave thermoablation in patients with obstructive benign prostatic hyperplasia: a phase I clinical study with a new mini-choked microwave applicator. *J Endourol.* Jul 2008;22(7):1509-1517.
[42] Zargar Shoshtari MA, Mirzazadeh M, Banai M, Jamshidi M, Mehravaran K. Radiofrequency-induced thermotherapy in benign prostatic hyperplasia. *Urol J.* Winter 2006;3(1):44-48.
[43] El-Husseiny T, Buchholz N. Transurethral ethanol ablation of the prostate for symptomatic benign prostatic hyperplasia: long-term follow-up. *J Endourol.* Mar 2011;25(3):477-480.
[44] Leocadio DE, Frenkl TL, Stein BS. Office based transurethral needle ablation of the prostate with analgesia and local anesthesia. *J Urol.* Nov 2007;178(5):2052-2054; discussion 2054.
[45] Pedersen JM, Romundstad PR, Mjones JG, Arum CJ. 2-year followup pressure flow studies of prostate photoselective vaporization using local anesthesia with sedation. *J Urol.* Apr 2009;181(4):1794-1799.
[46] Shinohara K, Roach M, 3rd. Technique for implantation of fiducial markers in the prostate. *Urology.* Feb 2008;71(2):196-200.
[47] Linden RA, Weiner PR, Gomella LG, et al. Technique of outpatient placement of intraprostatic fiducial markers before external beam radiotherapy. *Urology.* Apr 2009;73(4):881-886.
[48] Wallner K. Prostate brachytherapy under local anesthesia; lessons from the first 600 patients. *Brachytherapy.* 2002;1(3):145-148.
[49] Hirsch IH. Integrative urology: a spectrum of complementary and alternative therapy. *Urology.* Aug 1 2000;56(2):185-189.
[50] Inal G, Yazici S, Adsan O, Ozturk B, Kosan M, Centinkaya M. Effect of periprostatic nerve blockade before transrectal ultrasound-guided prostate biopsy on patient comfort: a randomized placebo controlled study. *International journal of urology : official journal of the Japanese Urological Association.* 2004;11(3):148-151.
[51] Richman JM, Carter HB, Hanna MN, et al. Efficacy of periprostatic local anesthetic for prostate biopsy analgesia: a meta-analysis. *Urology.* Jun 2006;67(6):1224-1228.

[52] Hergan L, Kashefi C, Parsons JK. Local anesthetic reduces pain associated with transrectal ultrasound-guided prostate biopsy: a meta-analysis. *Urology.* Mar 2007;69(3):520-525.
[53] Tiong HY, Liew LC, Samuel M, Consigliere D, Esuvaranathan K. A meta-analysis of local anesthesia for transrectal ultrasound-guided biopsy of the prostate. *Prostate Cancer Prostatic Dis.* 2007;10(2):127-136.
[54] Song SH, Kim JK, Song K, Ahn H, Kim CS. Effectiveness of local anaesthesia techniques in patients undergoing transrectal ultrasound-guided prostate biopsy: a prospective randomized study. *Int J Urol.* Jun 2006;13(6):707-710.
[55] Akan H, Yildiz O, Dalva I, Yucesoy C. Comparison of two periprostatic nerve blockade techniques for transrectal ultrasound-guided prostate biopsy: bilateral basal injection and single apical injection. *Urology.* Jan 2009;73(1):23-26.
[56] Kuppusamy S, Faizal N, Quek KF, Razack AH, Dublin N. The efficacy of periprostatic local anaesthetic infiltration in transrectal ultrasound biopsy of prostate: a prospective randomised control study. *World J Urol.* Dec 2010;28(6):673-676.
[57] Ozden E, Yaman O, Gogus C, Ozgencil E, Soygur T. The optimum doses of and injection locations for periprostatic nerve blockade for transrectal ultrasound guided biopsy of the prostate: a prospective, randomized, placebo controlled study. *J Urol.* Dec 2003;170(6 Pt 1):2319-2322.
[58] Lee-Elliott CE, Dundas D, Patel U. Randomized trial of lidocaine vs lidocaine/bupivacaine periprostatic injection on longitudinal pain scores after prostate biopsy. *The Journal of urology.* Jan 2004;171(1):247-250.
[59] Yurdakul T, Taspinar B, Kilic O, Kilinc M, Serarslan A. Topical and long-acting local anesthetic for prostate biopsy: a prospective randomized placebo-controlled study. *Urologia internationalis.* 2009;83(2):151-154.
[60] Obek C, Ozkan B, Tunc B, Can G, Yalcin V, Solok V. Comparison of 3 different methods of anesthesia before transrectal prostate biopsy: a prospective randomized trial. *J Urol.* Aug 2004;172(2):502-505.
[61] Skriapas K, Konstantinidis C, Samarinas M, Xanthis S, Gekas A. Comparison between lidocaine and glyceryl trinitrate ointment for perianal-intrarectal local anesthesia before transrectal ultrasonography-guided prostate biopsy: a pacebo-controlled trial. *Urology.* 2011;77(4):905-908.
[62] Raber M, Scattoni V, Roscigno M, et al. Topical prilocaine-lidocaine cream combined with peripheral nerve block improves pain control in prostatic biopsy: results from a prospective randomized trial. *Eur Urol.* May 2008;53(5):967-973.
[63] Giannarini G, Autorino R, Valent F, et al. Combination of perianal-intrarectal lidocaine-prilocaine cream and periprostatic nerve block for pain control during transrectal ultrasound guided prostate biopsy: a randomized, controlled trial. *J Urol.* Feb 2009;181(2):585-591; discussion 591-583.
[64] Mutaguchi K, Shinohara K, Matsubara A, Yasumoto H, Mita K, Usui T. Local anesthesia during 10 core biopsy of the prostate: comparison of 2 methods. *J Urol.* Mar 2005;173(3):742-745.
[65] Ashley RA, Inman BA, Routh JC, et al. Preventing pain during office biopsy of the prostate: a single center, prospective, double-blind, 3-arm, parallel group, randomized clinical trial. *Cancer.* Oct 15 2007;110(8):1708-1714.

[66] Binggian L, Peihuan L, Yudong W, Jinxing W, Zhiyong W. Intraprostatic local anesthesia with periprostatic nerve block for transrectal ultrasound guided prostate biopsy. *The Journal of urology.* 2009;182(2):479-483.

[67] Cam K, Sener M, Kayikci A, Akman Y, Erol A. Combined periprostatic and intraprostatic local anesthesia for prostate biopsy: a double-blind, placebo controlled, randomized trial. *J Urol.* Jul 2008;180(1):141-144; discussion 144-145.

[68] Lee HY, Lee HJ, Byun SS, Lee SE, Hong SK, Kim SH. Effect of intraprostatic local anesthesia during transrectal ultrasound guided prostate biopsy: comparison of 3 methods in a randomized, double-blind, placebo controlled trial. *J Urol.* Aug 2007;178(2):469-472; discussion 472.

[69] Turgut AT, Olcucuoglu E, Kosar P, Geyik PO, Kosar U. Complications and limitations related to periprostatic local anesthesia before TRUS-guided prostate biopsy. *J Clin Ultrasound.* Feb 2008;36(2):67-71.

[70] Obek C, Onal B, Ozkan B, Onder AU, Yalcin V, Solok V. Is periprostatic local anesthesia for transrectal ultrasound guided prostate biopsy associated with increased infectious or hemorrhagic complications? A prospective randomized trial. *J Urol.* Aug 2002;168(2):558-561.

[71] Cormio L, Lorusso F, Selvaggio O, et al. Noninfiltrative anesthesia for transrectal prostate biopsy: A randomized prospective study comparing lidocaine-prilocaine cream and lidocaine-ketorolac gel. *Urol Oncol.* Mar 9 2011.

[72] Raaijmakers R, Kirkels WJ, Roobol MJ, Wildhagen MF, Schrder FH. Complication rates and risk factors of 5802 transrectal ultrasound-guided sextant biopsies of the prostate within a population-based screening program. *Urology.* Nov 2002;60(5):826-830.

[73] Taverna G, Maffezzini M, Benetti A, Seveso M, Giusti G, Graziotti P. A single injection of lidocaine as local anesthesia for ultrasound guided needle biopsy of the prostate. *J Urol.* Jan 2002;167(1):222-223.

[74] Addla SK, Adeyoju AA, Wemyss-Holden GD, Neilson D. Local anaesthetic for transrectal ultrasound-guided prostate biopsy: a prospective, randomized, double blind, placebo-controlled study. *Eur Urol.* May 2003;43(5):441-443.

6

Achilles Tendon Repair Under Local Anesthesia

Andrej Čretnik
University Clinical Centre Maribor, Department of Traumatology
Slovenia

1. Introduction

Achilles tendon rupture is not a very common injury, but it has always attracted a great attention. Hippocrates is believed to first write about its treatment, but the first description of the Achilles tendon rupture can be found in the works of Ambrois Pare in 1575 (Bradley & Tibone, 1990; Maffulli, 1999).

Despite many different studies and metaanalyses, there is no universal agreement about the optimal management strategy of acute total Achilles tendon rupture. Most authors prefer open surgical repair as it contributes to a low incidence of re-rupture, ranging from 1,4% to 2,8% (Cetti et al., 1993; Inglis & Sculco, 1981; Lo et al., 1997; Maffulli, 1999; Thermann & Zwipp, 1989; Wills et al. 1986). Strong repair with the restored length and optional augmentation offers the possibility of early functional treatment (Carter et al., 1992). As it is associated with significant number of complications (11,8% to 21,6%) as well as high costs, some authors advocate conservative treatment (Cetti et al., 1993; Kocher et al., 2002; Lea & Smith, 1972; McComis et al., 1997; Nistor, 1981; Wills et al. 1986). High incidence of reruptures (12% to 17%), lengthened tendon and loss of strength are the main arguments for the opponents to criticize this method (Cetti et al., 1993; Inglis et al., 1976; Inglis & Sculco, 1981; Kocher et al., 2002; Lo et al., 1997; Maffulli, 1999; Wills et al. 1986, Washburn et al., 1992, Webb & Bannister, 1999). There are more and more papers favouring functional conservative treatment, what can yield to better results according to the lower re-rupture rate and better functional results (Kangas et al., 2003; McComis et al., 1997; Thermann et al., 1995; Twaddle & Poon, 2007; Willits et al., 2010).

Percutaneous repair (first described by Ma & Griffith in 1977) seems to bridge the gap, combining the advantages of conservative and operative treatment (Assal et al., 2002; Bradley & Tibone, 1990; Buchgraber & Pässler 1997; Čretnik et al., 2004, 2005; Fitzgibbons et al., 1993; Lim et al., 2001). It has been criticised to be weaker than open repair (Hockenbury & Johns 1990) and with higher re-rupture rate (Webb & Bannister 1999). Biomechanical studies have shown significantly greater biomechanical strength of the proposed modified method (Čretnik et al. 2000), with the strength comparable to open procedures (Čretnik et al. 2000, Watson et al. 1999, Zandbergen et al. 2005). According to the significantly stronger repair functional postoperative treatment should be encouraged and as it can be performed in an outpatient manner and under local anesthesia there are almost no contraindications to the method (except hypersensitivity to lidocain) (Čretnik et al. 2004, 2005, 2010).

2. Tendon repair

2.1 Position & material

The procedure is performed with the patient prone and with the injured foot lying free on a table with the enabled manipulation of the foot from the neutral position to the maximal plantar flexion (see Figure 1). Regular cleaning and desinfection procedures are performed during pre-operative preparations.

In general 20 - 30 mililiters of lidocaine (without noradrenaline!) in a sterile syringe with a regular infiltration needle is used. No tourniquet is needed. Regularly no antibiotic or antithrombotic prophylaxis is given.

Resorbable thread - Vicryl (polyglactin) No.2, length at least 50 cm (Ethicon, Sommerville, New Jersey) on long (up to 15 cm) semicurved (could be also straight or specially bent), at the end triangularly cut needles (HeliPro, Jesenice, Slovenia) is used (see Figure 2). Usually any other long needle can be used – the procedure can be performed more conveniently with two needles (at each end of the thread), otherwise the needle must be swapped from one end of the thread to another.

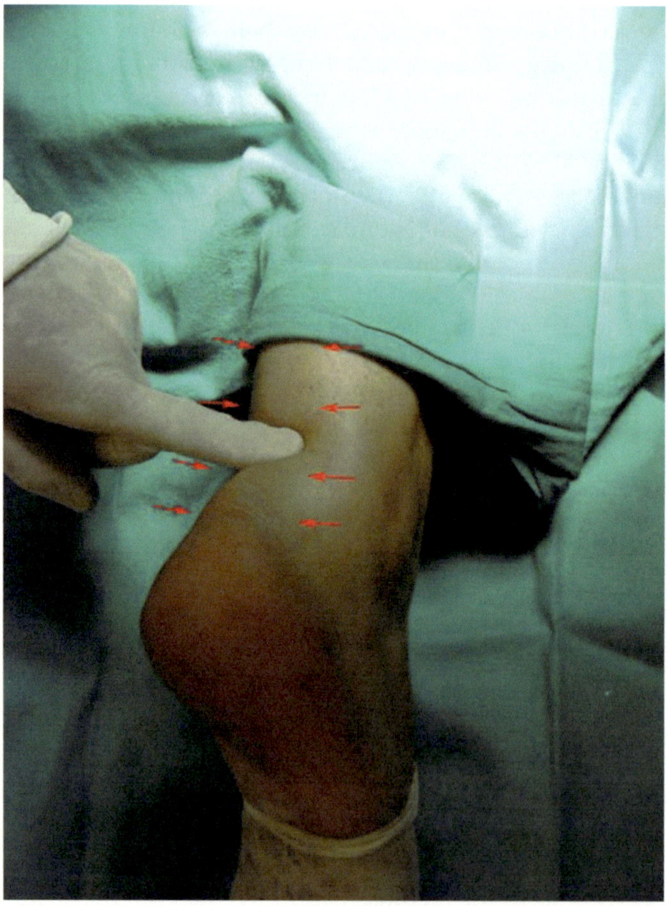

Fig. 1. (Palpating the gap)

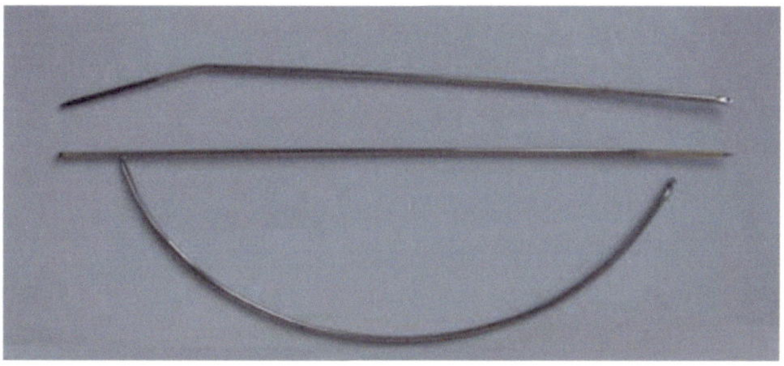

Fig. 2. (Needles)

2.2 Operative technique

Before starting, the rupture and diastasis (gap) must be localized (see Figure 1). After that, proximally (about five cm) and distally (about four cm) around the palpated gap, the cutis, subcutis and peritendineum are infiltrated at the marked points on the Figure 1. (see also Figure 3) All together there are eight puncture holes where the thread is later led. No other medications, nerve blocks or other types of anesthetics are given.

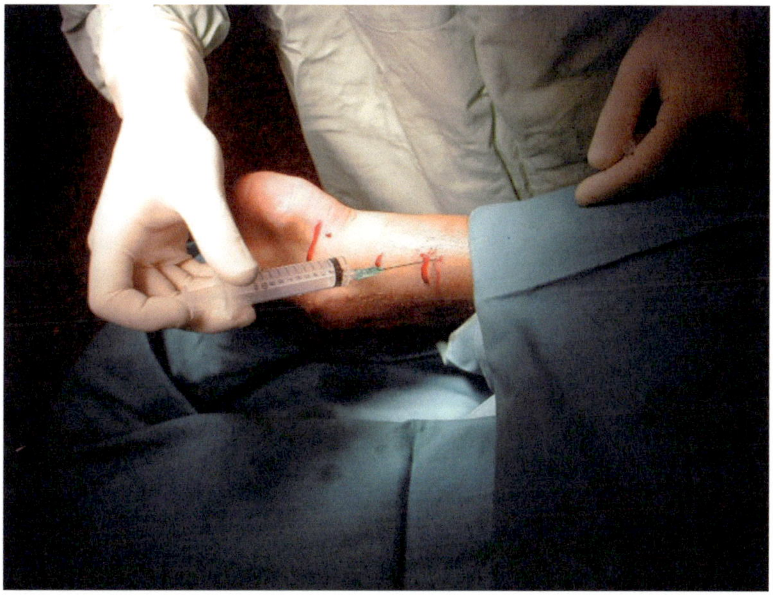

Fig. 3. (Infiltration with lidocaine)

Special attention must be paid to the lateral side, particularly proximally, where nervus suralis lies in the vicinity of the Achilles tendon and crosses it. According to the study of Citak et al. (2007) the lateral crossing of the sural nerve lies 8,7 - 12,4 cm proximally from the tuber calcanei. So the infiltration hole at the lateral side more than 9 cm proximally must not cross the lateral edge of Achilles tendon (it should lie even a little towards the inner area). Beside this, all the patient must be warned to report if any changes or sore pain are felt in this (nervus suralis) area during the puncture or infiltration. In that case, the puncture site must be moved for about half of or one cm towards the middle (the inner side) what can help to avoid sural nerve entrapment. In order to avoid direct sural nerve lesion and patient's comfort thinner infiltration needle (24-25 gauge) along with gentle injection could be used.

The procedure is started and finished medially and distally. First, the suture on the long, semicurved needle is transversely passed through the tendon (see scheme **a** on Figure 4), proceeding with the cross (diagonal) suture (see scheme **b** on Figure 4). If two needles (at each end of the thread) are used there is no need of swapping the needle from one end of

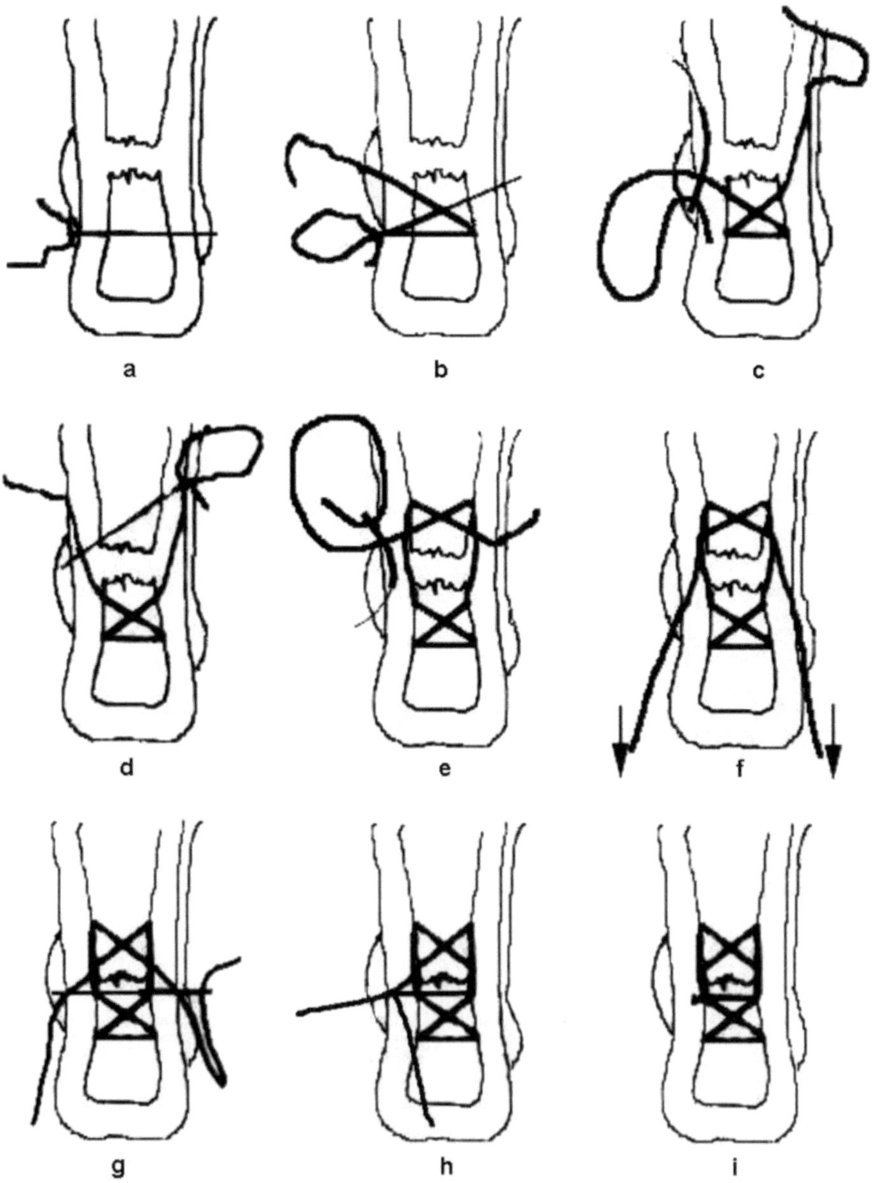

Fig. 4. (Scheme - from Journal of Foot and Ankle Surgery, 2004)

the thread to another and if the needles are used simultaneously (the first left thrusted in untill the second passes it) no hitting or cutting the thread during the cross could occur (in this way only the metal (needle) can be hit). At every site of the first needle entrance or exit, the incision should be widened in longitudinal direction by pushing the scalpel blade (No.11) on the thrust-in needle to enable the surgeon to sink the thread subcutaneously (on the paratenon) when proceeding the suture through the same hole (see Figure 5). A small haemostat can also be used to widen the hole and enable the sinking of the thread through the same hole.

It is useful to always pull each side of the thread in a zig-zag manner after exiting each hole, so the thread can really slide and enable approximation of the torn ends at the end of the procedure. The thread is then led longitudinally, subcutaneously - extratendineously (see scheme **c** on Figure 4) and the next cross through the tendon is done proximally (see scheme **d** on Figure 4). After that, both ends are led extratendineously back through the third and second hole distally (see scheme **e** on Figure 4) and pulled symmetrically back with feeling until both ends of the torn Achilles tendon are completely approximated and the defect is no longer palpable (see scheme **f** on Figure 4).

After approximating the torn Achilles tendon ends, the lateral end of the thread is passed medially (see scheme **g** on Figure 4) (both ends of the thread must be held tightened at that time) where, after final tightening, the suture is tied (see scheme **h** on Figure 4). The knots are sunk (buried) subcutaneously through the previously widened second medial stab wound distally (see scheme **i** on Figure 4). At the end nothing can be seen on the surface, except eight small stab wounds and the folds of skin that later completely disappear (see Figure 6). Small stab wounds can be closed with very fine sutures but this is routinely not performed (Cretnik et al. 2004, 2005, 2010).

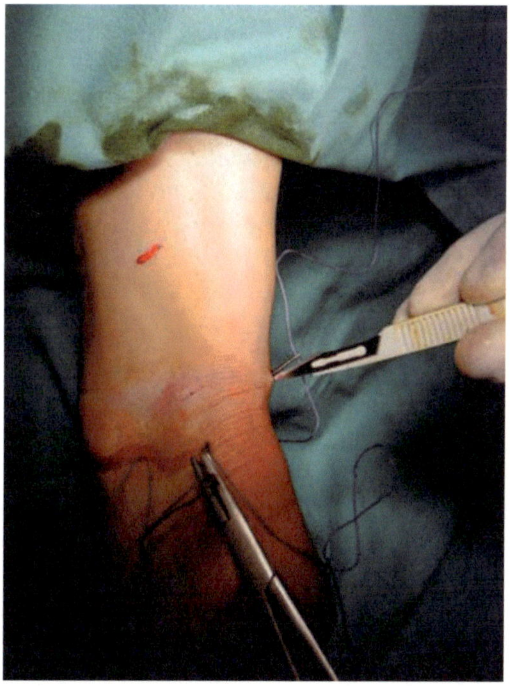

Fig. 5. (Widening the hole with blade No. 11)

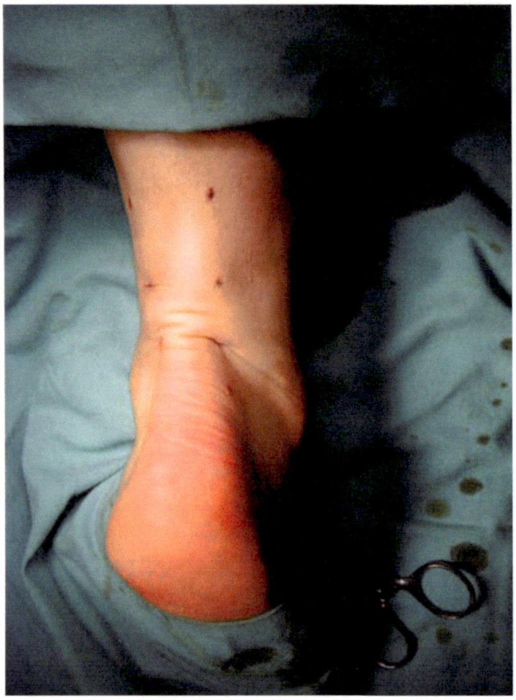

Fig. 6. (Final outlook)

Approximation can be intra- and postoperatively controlled by ultrasonography - transducer is simply put into the sterile glove (or standard protection cover for arthroscopy) with the use of sterile gel or lidocaine gel (regularly used in urology). If any gap between the torn ends persists they should be pulled together with both ends of the thread further before the suture is tied (foot should be positioned in the maximal plantar flexion). Before final tightening it's very useful to gently manipulate with the foot in plantar and dorsal direction, so the thread can really be sunk at the surface of the tendon and the approximated ends secured with the tensioned thread without any loops or soft tissue captured. In the majority of cases disappearing of the gap and good approximation can be easily palpated but in the first cases until some experience is gained or if any doubt about that persist it's very helpful to use the ultrasonographic control.

2.3 Postoperative procedure

After the procedure, sterile dressing and a cast splint at the dorsal part with the foot in about 20 degrees of plantar flexion is applied. The first re-dressing is done the second day, when a functional orthosis made from softcast and stockinette is regularly applied for three weeks with the foot in about 20 degrees of plantar flexion (see Figure 7 and 8). It enables immediate plantar flexion and thus functional treatment with easy dressings and removal for hygienic procedures (washing). Patients should use crutches to walk and a careful weightbearing of approximately 5 kg is immediately allowed. In next three weeks progressive weightbearing up to 20 kg is allowed. No special heel or any special shoes are routinely used, although they can make walking easier (with supported heel).

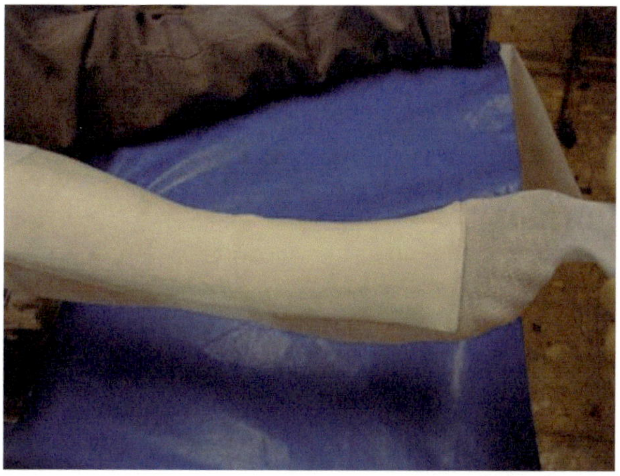

Fig. 7. (Softcast functional orthosis - preparation with stockinette)

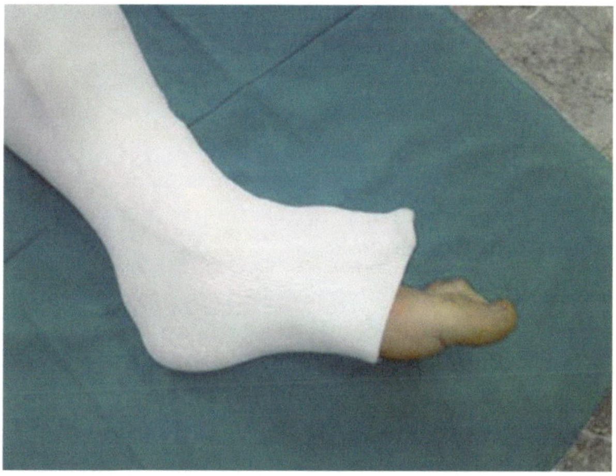

Fig. 8. (plantar flexion in orthosis)

After three weeks a new immobilization with the foot in neutral position (zero degrees of dorsiflexion) is applied. It's made in the same way to enable plantar flexion of the foot and to prevent dorsiflexion. It can also be made of cast, but softcast is much more convenient, lighter and water resistant. Patients keep walking with crutches and are allowed to bear weight as tolerated. They may walk with orthosis without crutches if they are able to and have no pain.

According to the principle of better healing if the ends are always sligthly tensioned, orthosis can be changed after two and four weeks and plantar flexion gradually diminished from 20 degrees to 10 degrees and at four weeks to zero degrees. If patients are walking with crutches and encouraged to gradually increase weightbearing, diminishing of plantar flexion to neutral position can be achieved with the softcast orthosis spontaneously, as it is becoming slowly more and more soften and allows reaching neutral position in four weeks without any change of orthosis and thus number of scheduled visits at clinics (and costs) can be further reduced.

After six weeks the immobilization (orthosis) is removed and the patients are allowed to walk (without crutches) and start with careful rehabilitation until pain is felt (motion exercises, bathing, progressive resistance exercises, loads with elastic band …). A special attention should be given to the correct pattern of walking (without limping). The patients are encouraged to start swimming and walking in the pool with weightbearing as much as tolerated in water. Stretching exercises are routinely allowed after eight weeks with careful increasing of the load. Raising on toes or heels is allowed twelve weeks after the operation and limited sports activities individually after three months with recommended full loading six months after operation. Indeed, many patients are starting with such activities(much) earlier with no complaints.

2.4 Discussion

There are many percutaneous closed (Čretnik et al., 2000, 2004, 2005; Gorschewsky et al., 2004; Ma & Griffith, 1977; Majewsky et al., 2006; Webb & Bannister, 1999) and semi-open methods (Amlang et al., 2006; Assal et al, 2002; Kakiuchi, 1995) proposed. They are four or six stab – incision techniques with one-aside pulling technique and consequently arose problem with non or malaligned stumps (so called fish-tail phenomenon) (Hockenbury & Johns, 1990)). The proposed method, described above (Čretnik et al. 2004, 2005, 2010), is the only (at the moment) eight stab-incision technique and the only one with symmetrical pulling of both sides of the torn end, using double pulley principle, what enables appropriate adaptation without "fish- tail" phenomenon and with significantly reduced pulling - force needed. It enables also ultrasonographic control ad thus objectively confirmed approximation of the torn ends.

Biomechanical studies have confirmed significantly stronger repair with the proposed method in comparison to other percutaneous methods and comparable results to the open methods (Assal et al., 2002, Čretnik et al., 2000, Hockenbury & Johns, 1990, Watson et al., 1995, Zandbergen et al., 2005). The ultimate load failure force with the open Kessler technique with two strands of Ethibond No. 1 was 85 N and with the Bunnell technique with the same strands was 93 N. The ultimate load failure with the percutaneous Ma and Griffith technique with one strand of Vicryl No.2 was 111 N and with the proposed method (Čretnik et al. 2000) with the same material was 214 N. The ultimate load failure with the open Krackow Locking Loop with 4 strands of Ethibond No. 1 was 147 N and with 4 strands of Ethibond No. 2 222 N. The strongest repair in human testing models was achieved with the open triple bundle technique with 6 strands of Ethibond No 1 (453N). The results showed comparable results of the proposed method with one resorbable strand of Vicryl No.2 to open repair with the 4 strands of non-resorbable Ethibond No.1 with the Krackow Locking Loop technique (Čretnik et al., 2000,. Watson et al., 1995, Zandbergen et al., 2005).

The adequacy of apposition and fixation of torn ends seems to be crucial with all the methods and techniques. Complete rupture leads to retraction of the triceps surae and consequently to diastasis of the torn ends. As with conservative treatment the torn ends of the tendon stay apart (at the beginning in many cases good adaptation can be achieved with plantar flexion of the foot but the retraction occurs in next days, pulling torn ends apart and making diastasis), this brings the tendon to heal in the lengthened position and leads to the loss of normal tone and a weakening of the musculature (Čretnik et al., 2005, Inglis et al., 1976, Washburn et al., 1992). The gap is filled with fibrous tissue that is never as strong as the original tendon, contributing to a high incidence of rerupture (Webb & Bannister, 1999; Wills et al., 1986). The review studies with a large number of patients show the rerupture rate with conservative treatment of 12% (Webb & Bannister, 1999; Lo et al., 1997) to 13,4% (Cetti et al., 1993) although there could be found reports on the functional conservative treatment with the lower incidence of the rerupture rate (Kangas et al., 2003; McComis et al., 1997; Thermann et al., 1995; Twaddle & Poon, 2007; Willits et al., 2010).

Open repair enables the best visualization and adaptation of the torn ends and the possibility of augmentation with different types of strips and tendon parts to reduce the number of reruptures to minimum. It must be stressed that many times the approximation of the torn ends could not be achieved easy with open and particularly with percutaneous repair (Čretnik et al., 2005). The torn ends are often extremely friable and not as even, as we like to believe and there are many times difficulties to pull together the torn ends and achieve a good and firm adaptation, particularly using the techniques with simple loop or modified Bunnell's sutures (Buchgraber & Pässler 1997; Ma & Griffith, 1977; Webb & Bannister, 1999). As shown in biomechanical studies above there are big differences in the strength of repair and consequently in the resistance ability during the healing process, particularly if functional treatment with the persistent tension to the torn ends is chosen. It is worth to be stressed therefore to choose the strongest method as possible. Stronger repair with good approximation of the torn ends provides healing with no elongation, low amount of the fibrous tissue, more resistance in functional postoperative treatment and thus low number of re-rupture rate.

Personal experience with the analysis of the percutaneously treated patients under local anesthesia in the period from 1991 to 2006 revealed 270 operated on and 267 finally analyzed patients (98,8%) with 8 (2,96%) re-ruptures (partial or complete) with only two patients needed to be re- operated on in an open way because of the diastasis of torn ends (the others were treated conservatively with ultrasonographic control and cast in plantar flexion for three weeks and additional three weeks in neutral position) with good final result in all cases (of re-ruptures) with no major or minor complications and with 216 patients (80,8%) who returned to previous activities.

Percutaneous method is criticized to be a closed (blind) one, where the exact position of the torn ends and approximation cannot be visualized (Maffulli, 1999). Semi-open method was proposed as a solution, where (small) incision is made at the site of rupture and the approximation is checked under visual control (Kakiuchi, 1995). Special instruments were developed for this method (Achillon®), Dresdner instrument), so the sural nerve injuries were almost completely reduced (Amlang et al, 2006; Assal et al. 2002;). Opening the site of a rupture the injury becomes an open one with all the risks and loss of haematoma with stimulating factors (mediators) (Growth Factors, Platelet Rich Plasma...) (Čretnik et al. 2005). However, as the torn ends are pulled apart, the gap between them can be palpated and the position of the ends thereby located. Addition of ultrasonography presents a precise tool for diagnosing the rupture and locating the gap and torn ends and control of approximation, what can be usually also clinically palpated (Čretnik et al, 2005). In our series with ultrasonographic control diastasis after the operation never exceeded 0,5 cm (Čretnik et al, 2005) what has been considered as an acceptable one in functional conservative treatment (Thermann & Zwipp, 1989, Thermann et al., 1995).

Prospective study has shown significiantly fewer major and total number of complications in the group of proposed percutaneous repairs in comparison with the group of open repairs. There were slightly more reruptures and sural nerve disturbances in the group of percutaneous repairs with no statistically significant difference. Functional assessment using various scores showed no statistically significant differences between both groups (Čretnik et al., 2005).

2.5 Conclusion

Proposed modified technique under local anesthesia seems probably more demanding but can be performed with the careful adherence to the instructions (particulars). It is very important to approximate the torn ends enough, so that the defect is clinically no longer palpable. Plantar flexion of the foot during reapproximation assists in this maneuver. Functional postoperative treatment with the simple softcast removable brace should be encouraged in all the operated on patients.

Long term results support the choice of the proposed modified percutaneous method under local anesthesia as the method that brings comparable functional results to open repair, with a significantly lower rate of complications.

3. References

Amlang, M.H.; Christiani, P.; Heinz, P. & Zwipp, H. (2006). The percutaneous Suture of the Achilles Tendon with the Dresden Instrument. *Operative Orthopädie und Traumatologie.* Vol.18, No.4., pp. 287-299

Assal, M.; Jung, M.; Stern, R.; Rippstein, P.; Delmi, M. & Hoffmeyer, P. (2002). Limited open repair of Achilles tendon ruptures. A technique with a new instrument and findings of a prospective multicenter study. *J Bone Joint Surg* 84A:161-170

Bradley, J.P. & Tibone, J.E. (1990). Percutaneous and open surgical repairs of Achilles tendon ruptures. A comparative study. *Am J Sports Med,* 18: 188-195

Buchgraber, A. & Pässler, H.H. (1997). Percutaneous repair of Achilles tendon rupture. Immobilization versus functional postoperative treatment. *Clin Orthop* 341: 113-122

Carter TR, Fowler PJ, Blokker C. (1992). Functional postoperative treatment of Achilles tendon repair. *Am J Sports Med* 20: 459-462

Cetti R, Christensen SE, Ejsted R, (1993) al: Operative versus nonoperative treatment of Achilles tendon rupture. *Am J Sports Med* 21: 791-799,

Citak, M.; Knoblach, K.; Albrecht, K.; Krettek, C. & Hufner T. (2007). Anatomy oft he sural nerve in a computer assisted model: implicationsfor surgical minimal-invasive Achilles tendon repair. *Br J Sports Med,* 41, 456-458

Čretnik, A; Žlajpah, L; Smrkolj, V. & Kosanović, M. (2000) The strength of percutaneous methods of repair of the Achilles tendon : a biomechanical study. Med. Sci. Sports Exerc. 32:16-20,.

Čretnik, A; Smrkolj, V. & Kosanović, M. (2004). Percutaneous suturing of the ruptured Achilles tendon under local anesthesia. *J. Foot Ankle Surg.* Vol.43, No.2., pp. 72-81

Čretnik, A; Smrkolj, V. & Kosanović, M. (2005). Percutaneous versus open repair of the ruptured Achilles tendon. A comparative study. *Am. J. Sports Med.* 33:1369-1379

Čretnik, A; Košir, R. & Kosanović, M. (2010) Incidence and outcome of operatively treated achilles tendon rupture in the elderly. *Foot ankle int.*, Vol. 31, No.1, pp 14-18

Fitzgibbons, R.E.; Hefferon, J. & Hill, J. (1993). Percutaneous Achilles tendon repair. *Am J Sports Med* 21: 724-727

Gorschewsky, O; Pitzl, M; Pütz, A; Klakow, A. & Neumann, W. (2004). Percutaneous repair of Acute Achilles Tendon Rupture. Foot Ankle Int. 25:219-224

Hockenbury, R.T. &, Johns, J.C. (1990). A biomechanical in vitro comparison of open versus percutaneous repair of tendon Achilles. *Foot Ankle Int* 11: 67-72,

Inglis, A.E.; Scott WN, Sculco TP. & Paterson, A.H. (1976). Ruptures of the tendon Achillis. An objective assessment of surgical and non-surgical treatment. *J Bone Joint Surg* 58A: 990-999

Inglis, A.E. & Sculco, T.P. (1981). Surgical repair of ruptures of the tendon Achillis. *Clin Orthop* 156: 160-169

Kakiuchi, M. (1995). A combined open and percutaneous technique for repair of tendon Achillis. Comparison with open repair. *J Bone Joint Surg* 77B: 60-63

Kangas, J.A.; Pajala, A.; Siira, P.; Hamalainen, M. & Leppilahti, J. (2003) Early functional treatment versus early immobilization in tension of the musculotendinous unit after Achilles rupture repair: a prospective randomized, clinical study. *J Trauma*, 54, 1171 - 1180

Kocher MS, Bishop J, Marshall R.; Briggs, K.K. & Hawkins, R.J. (2002): Operative versus Nonoperative Management of Acute Achilles Tendon Rupture. Expected-value Decision Analysis. *Am J Sports Med* 30: 783-790,

Lea, R.B. & Smith, L. (1972). Non-surgical treatment of tendon Achillis ruptures. *J Bone Joint Surg* 54A: 1398-1407,

Lim J, Dalal R, Waseem M. (2001). Percutaneous vs. Open repair of the Ruptured Achilles Tendon - A Prospective randomized Controlled Study. *Foot Ankle Int* 22: 559-568

Lo IK, Kirkley A, Nonweiler B. & Kumbhare, D.A. (1997). Operative versus nonoperative treatment of acute Achilles tendon ruptures: a quantitative review. *Clin J Sport Med*, 7: 207-211

Ma GWC, Griffith TG. (1977). Percutaneous repair of acute closed ruptured Achilles tendon: A new technique. *Clin Orthop* 128: 247-255,

Maffuli, N. (1999). Rupture of the Achilles tendon. *J Bone Joint Surg*, 81A: 1019-1036

Majewski, M.; Rohrbach, M.; Czaja, S. & Ochsner, P. (2006). Avoiding sural nerve injuries during percutaneous Achilles tendon repair. *Am J Sports Med*, Vol.34, No.5, pp. 793-798

McComis, G.P.; Nawoczenski, D.A. & DeHaven, K.E. (1997). Functional bracing for rupture of the Achilles tendon. Clinical results and analysis of ground-reaction forces and temporal data. *J Bone Joint Surg* 79A: 1799-1808

Nistor, L. (1981). Surgical and non-surgical treatment of Achilles tendon rupture. *A prospective randomized study. J Bone Joint Surg* 63A: 394-399,

Thermann, H. & Zwipp, H. (1989). Achillessehnenruptur. *Orthopäde* 18: 321-335,

Thermann, H.; Zwipp, H. & Tscherne, H. (1995). Functional treatment concept of acute rupture of the Achilles tendon. 2 years results of a prospective randomized study. *Unfallchirurg*, 98: 21 - 32

Twaddle, B. C. & Poon, P. (2007). Early motion for Achilles tendon ruptures: is surgery important? A randomized prospective study. *Am J Sports Med.* Vol.35, No.12, pp. 2033 - 2038

Washburn SD, Caiozzo VJ, Wills CA.; Hunt, B.J. & Prietto C.A. (1992). Alterations in the in-vivo torque-velocity relationship after Achilles tendon rupture. Further evidence of speed- specific impairment. *Clin Orthop* 279: 237-245

Watson, T.W.; Jurist, K.A.; Yang, K.H. & Shen, K.L. (1995). The strength of Achilles tendon repair: an in vitro study of the biomechanical behaviour in human cadaver tendons. *Foot Ankle Int.* 16, pp. 191-195

Webb, J.M. & Bannister, G.C. (1999). Percutaneous repair of the ruptured tendon Achillis. *J. Bone Joint Surg,* 81B: 877-880

Willits, K.; Amendola, A.; Bryant, D.; Mohtadi N. G.; Giffin, J.R.; Fowler, P.; Kean, C. O. & Kirkley, A. (2010). Operative versus nonoperative treatment of acute Achilles tendon ruptures: a multicenter randomized trial using accelerated functional rehabilitation. *J Bone Joint Surg Am.* Vol.92, No.17, pp. 2767-2775

Wills CA, Washburn S, Caiozzo V. & Prietto C.A. (1986). Achilles tendon rupture. A review of the literature comparing surgical versus nonsurgical treatment. *Clin Orthop* 207: 156-163

Zandbergen, R.A., de Boer, S.F.; Swiestra, B.A.; Day, J.; Kleinrensink, G.J. & Beumer, A. (2005). Surgical treatment of Achilles tendon rupture: examination of strength of 3 types of suture techniques in a cadaver model. *Acta Orthop.* 76, pp. 408-411

7

The Use of Topical Cream Anesthetics in Office Procedures of the External Genitalia

Kostis Gyftopoulos
Urologic Surgeon, Olympion Hospital and Department of Anatomy, University of Patras Greece

1. Introduction

The use of anesthesia during nineteenth century was extremely limited due to the hazards of the available anesthetics and the inability to successfully monitor the patient. This resulted in the majority of surgical procedures being performed without any anesthesia (Gordetsky et al, 2011). A revolutionary step in the history of anesthetics began in 1884, when Carl Koller, a scientist from Vienna, experimented with topical application of cocaine in the eye, achieving adequate surgical analgesia, without the potentially lethal side effects of inhalation anesthesia (Neilson, n.d.). The use of this natural alkaloid provided results superior to the contemporary general anesthesia and surgeons quickly appreciated the advantages of local anesthetics. Especially urologists embraced rapidly the promising local anesthetic and began experimenting with cocaine as a local agent for urological procedures, mainly by topical and intraurethral application (Gordetsky et al, 2011). It took a while for the initial enthusiasm to settle down as reports for side effects and addiction were bringing debate in the medical community. The need for less toxic drugs would lead to synthetic local drugs such as procaine; the discovery of the stable amide lignocaine in 1948 by Lofgren was an important milestone in the development of safe and effective local anesthetics.

A plethora of urological or gynecological surgical procedures are performed nowadays under local anesthesia at an office setting. In the male these minor procedures usually deal with the prepuce or the urethral meatus (separation of preputial adhesions, short frenulum plasty, meatotomy, modified or complete circumcision). In the female, these procedures deal with lesions of the vulvar skin or the cervix (vulvar or vaginal biopsy, laser treatment of vulvar and cervical lesions, hysteroscopy). Removal of genital warts (condylomata accuminata) is also a common procedure under local anesthesia in both genders. The need for some form of anesthesia is important for both the patient and the surgeon. For the patient it is a human right not to suffer pain or distress associated with a surgical procedure. On the other hand, withholding analgesia may affect the quality of the surgical outcome, as the patient's anxiety, reaction to pain and improper movement may complicate the surgeon's ability to perform a delicate procedure. This is especially true in the above mentioned procedures due to the unique sensitivity of the external genitalia.

The diverse innervation of the genital skin, especially the penile and clitoral prepuce, may account for the increased discomfort during procedures of the external genitalia in both sexes. The penile and vulvar skin and mucosal surfaces are highly sensitive to pain (Zilbert

2002, Cold &Taylor, 1999). The somatosensory innervation of the genitalia is complex and still under debate. The male prepuce receives branches from the dorsal nerve of the penis and branches of the perineal nerve. Some sensory pathways of the genital tract may even by-pass the spinal cord through the vagus nerve. Moreover, the genital skin and especially the prepuce is rich in encapsulated somatosensory receptors, which include Meissner's corpuscles, Vater-Pacinian corpuscles and Merkel cells. These extremely sensitive receptors are probably part of the erogenous function of the genital skin (Cold & Taylor, 1999). Additionally, free nerve endings account for the protopathic sensitivity i.e. crude, poorly localized feelings which however include pain. This complex pattern of innervation not only explains the high sensitivity of the genital region but also emphasizes the need for adequate anesthesia for the performance of surgical procedures.

The most common way of achieving anesthesia in the genital area is infiltration of a local agent. This is a logical option for the majority of the afore-mentioned procedures, as they are relatively superficial. Local infiltration obviates the need for sedation and the risks of other forms of anesthesia; however it can still cause discomfort to the patient. Injections of local anesthetics are painful by themselves, may worsen needle anxiety and increase pain perception (Kaweski, 2008). Moreover they may cause bleeding and distort the surgical area by development of oedema or haematoma. There is also the risk of inadvertent intravascular injection, especially when larger volume of anesthetic solution is used. Topical anesthetic creams may in some cases replace injected local anesthetics. They are much more "patient-friendly", as they eliminate needle fear and pain in the beginning of the procedure. It has been shown that by using a topical anesthetic cream the patient's anxiety and distress of the procedure itself are alleviated. This is also valuable in children, as the pain factor and the increased pain perception are overcome with the application of a topical cream (Kaweski, 2008).

We hereby describe our experience on the efficacy and safety of a topical anesthetic cream (EMLA, Eutectic Mixture of Local Anesthetics, 2.5% lidocaine and 2.5% prilocaine) as topical anesthetic in several office surgical procedures of the external genitalia in both males and females.

2. Patients and methods

During a period of 8 years (2003-2010) a total of 321 patients were subjected to minor surgery of the external genitalia at an office setting under local anesthesia. The range of procedures included: Separation of preputial adhesions in boys, complete circumcision for phimosis, short frenulum plasty, meatotomy, fulguration of genital warts (penile, vulvar), fulguration of urethral (meatal) warts and excision of urethral prolapse in women. The distribution of cases is described in Table 1.

All patients were offered to choose between infiltration with a local anaesthetic and application of a topical cream as a form of local analgesia. After detailed information was given, all patients opted for the topical cream application. Informed consent was obtained by those patients whose genitals were photographed for archival and scientific purposes.

In all cases the topical cream used was EMLA 5 gr (Eutectic Mixture of Local Anesthetics, 2.5% lidocaine and 2.5% prilocaine), AstraZeneca, Inc. The amount of cream used varied among individuals and procedures (see below). For the fulguration of genital warts, frenulum plasty and haemostasis during circumcision we used the Birtcher Hyfercator Plus™ (Birtcher Medical Systems Inc, Utica, NY), a high frequency device used for monoterminal fulguration at low power settings (7-10 Watts).

PROCEDURE	No	MALE	FEMALE	AGE (mean± SD)
Preputial adhesions	17	17		52 months ± 18.7
Circumcision	68	68		47.8yrs ± 24.7
Short frenulum	152	152		24.9 yrs ± 4.7
Meatotomy	12	12		56.1 yrs ± 28.4
Genital warts	48	42	6	23.9 yrs ± 3.3
Urethral warts	17	17		24.5 yrs ± 5.8
Urethral prolapse	7		7	74.8 yrs ± 6.5

Table 1. Distribution of patients according to surgical procedure.

2.1 Application method and surgical procedure

2.1.1 Separation of preputial adhesions

Separation of preputial adhesions was performed in 17 boys (mean age±SD: 52 months ± 18.7). The procedure was reserved only for boys with partial preputial adhesion and history of previous inflammation (balanoposthitis) or previous urinary tract infection. Patients with verbal ability were thoroughly informed of the procedure and reassured that they would feel no pain. A small amount of EMLA (0.5-1gr) was smeared inside the preputial sac using a cotton tip. Children were allowed to relax for 20 minutes in the waiting room for the anesthetic to act. The procedure was accomplished by gentle traction of the prepuce and concomitant separation of the adhesions using a fine haemostatic clamp (mosquito clamp). Special care was taken not to force the separation of the fused mucosa, in order to avoid bleeding and glanular excoriation. After completion of the procedure, a small quantity of povidone iodine cream was applied and the prepuce was pulled back to cover the glans. The young boys were kept for one hour in the waiting room for monitoring and dismissed after thorough consultation of the parents on possible adverse effects during the following hours. Parents were advised to start local hygiene with a mild soap on the next day, gently retracting the foreskin. No further antiseptics or antibiotics were prescribed.

2.1.2 Short frenulum plasty

Short frenulum plasty was performed in 152 young males (mean age±SD: 24.9 yrs ± 4.7). The method used for short frenulum correction was the "pull and burn method" described previously (Gyftopoulos, 2009). Briefly, a small amount of EMLA cream (max 2 gr) was applied at the frenulum area and an occlusive dressing (Tegaderm®, 3M Inc.) was used to prevent the cream from leaking. After 20 minutes the adhesive dressing was gently removed, excess cream was cleaned, the glans was smeared with povidone iodine and the procedure started if the patient reported no pain at all at pinprick. By retracting the glans upwards, the point of maximum tension on the frenulum was noted (Fig. 1). A small horizontal cut was made using the Hyfercator and the superficial layer of the frenulum was gradually separated by applying gentle and stable traction to the glans and the shaft of the penis. Minor bleeders were sealed by the Hyfercator at low power, taking care not to severe the frenular artery that was now lying at the frenular bed. When full relaxation of the frenular chordee was achieved a small quantity of povidone iodine cream was applied on site and the prepuce was pulled back to cover the glans. Patients were instructed to start personal hygiene on the following day, with emphasis on keeping the trauma as dry as possible (e.g. by retracting the foreskin when voiding). No antibiotics were given and sexual abstinence was suggested for at least 15 days.

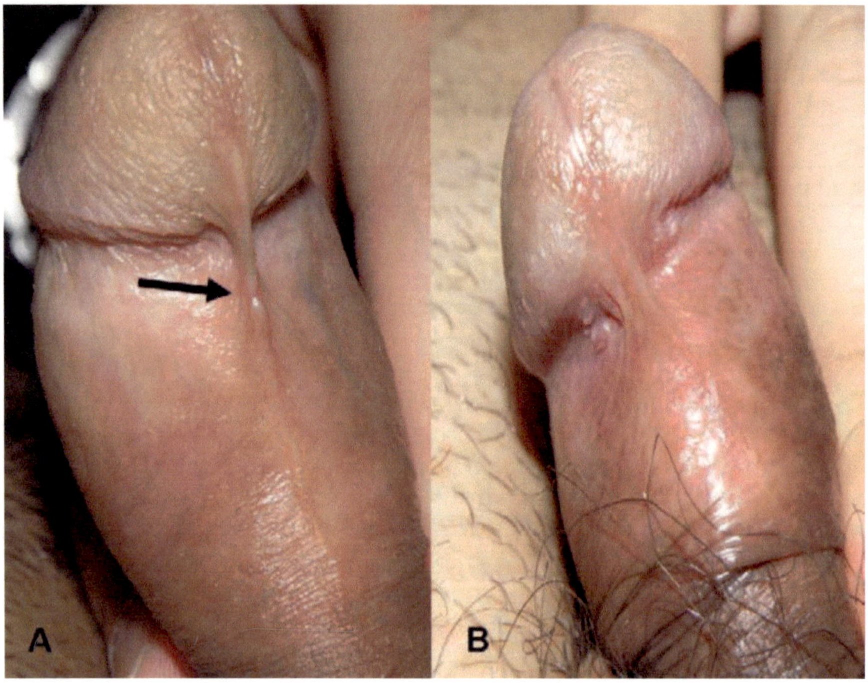

Fig. 1. Short frenulum cases. Note previous scar from trauma in case A (arrow).

2.1.3 Meatotomy

A total of 12 patients (mean age±SD: 56.1 yrs ± 28.4) were subjected to meatotomy due to meatal stenosis. In four cases the patient had Balanitis Xerotica Obliterans (BXO) affecting the glans and the meatus. A small quantity of EMLA cream (~1 gr) was applied using a small 1 ml syringe. An occlusive dressing (Tegaderm®, 3M Inc.) was used to prevent the cream from leaking. After 20 minutes the adhesive dressing was gently removed, the glans was squeezed to remove excess cream and a small haemostatic clip was used to spread the urethral meatus. An incision was made to the ventral surface of the meatus using the lancet of the Birtcher Hyfercator. The incision was extended ventrally (6 o'clock position) until a sufficient opening of the meatus was achieved. This was calibrated using the tip of a 18 Fr Tiemann catheter. In 4 patients the urethral mucosa was sutured at the meatal lips at the 3 and 9 o'clock position using fine absorbable sutures (5-0 polyglycolic acid, Safil Quick™, B. Braun Melsungen AG). No postoperative analgesia was given. The patients were advised to avoid irritative food and liquids (e.g. pepperoni, alcohol consumption) for the following days. Local hygiene (mild soap and water) was allowed from the following day.

2.1.4 Fulguration of urethral warts

A total of 17 male patients (mean age±SD: 24.5 yrs ± 5.8) were treated for warts (HPV lesions, condylomata acuminata) at the external urethral meatus. The lesions were limited to the meatus or fossa navicularis. A small quantity of EMLA cream (~1 gr) was applied using a small 1 ml syringe (Fig. 2). An occlusive dressing (Tegaderm®, 3M Inc.) was again used to prevent the cream from leaking. 20 minutes later the adhesive dressing was removed, the glans was squeezed to remove excess cream and a small haemostatic clip was used to spread the urethral meatus. The warts were fulgurated using the Birtcher Hyfercator at low power settings (approximately 5 Watts). In 7 cases (41%) there were multiple HPV lesions (up to three) inside the urethral meatus. All of these lesions were treated in one session.Suspicious reddish areas of the urethral mucosa, when present, were also fulgurated; however care was taken to limit the fulgurated area to approximately 40% of the mucosal surface in order to avoid possible meatal stenosis. In 5 cases a modified meatotomy was necessary in order to have access to the lesions. No postoperative analgesia was given. The patients were advised to consume at least 2 liters of clear water daily, to avoid irritative food and liquids (e.g. pepperoni, alcohol consumption, acidic refreshments) and to void frequently for the following week. Local hygiene (mild soap and water) was allowed from the following day but sexual abstinence was advised for at least 10 days; condom use was suggested after that period. The patients were also advised to inspect the meatal opening for possible recurrence during the healing period.

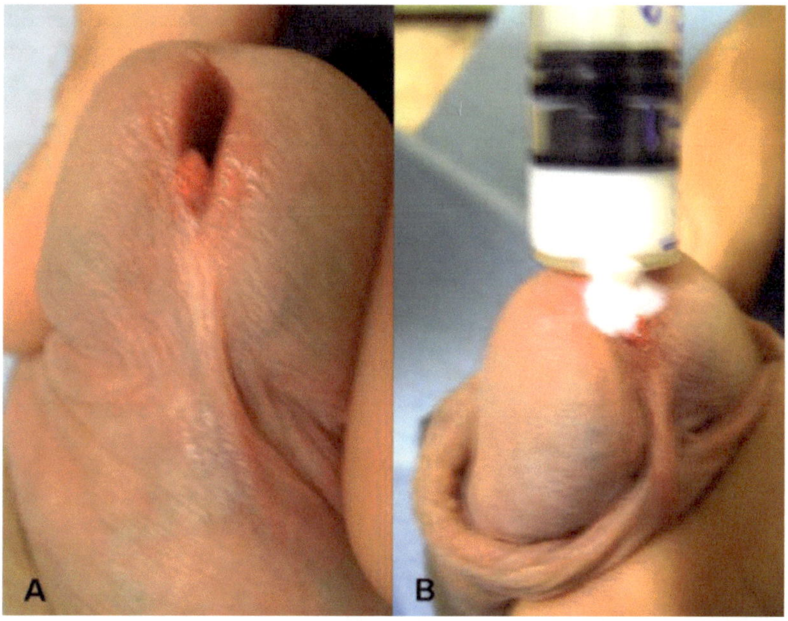

Fig. 2. HPV lesion protruding from the urethral meatus (A). Topical cream applied with a syringe (B).

2.1.5 Urethral prolapse correction

Seven elderly female patients (mean age±SD: 74.8 yrs ± 6.5), presenting with urethral prolapse were treated under topical anesthesia. After preparation of the genitalia with povidone iodine, the EMLA cream (approximately 2 gr) was applied inside the urethral mucosa using a small 5 ml syringe. The external meatus and parameatal tissue was also smeared with a small quantity of cream. No dressing was used but the patient was left in lithotomy position for 20 minutes. Subsequently the excess cream was removed, the prolapsed mucosa was grasped with an Allis forceps and the Birtcher Hyfercator was used to cut the prolapsed mucosa. Any bleeding vessels were sealed at the same time. After excision of the redundant mucosa, the mucosal edges were sutured to the meatus using fine absorbable sutures (4-0 polyglycolic acid, Safil QuickTM, B. Braun Melsungen AG) at the 3, 6, 9 and 12 o'clock positions. A 12 Fr Foley catheter was left in place for 24 hrs and the patient was advised to refrain from spicy food and alcohol consumption for the following 10 days.

2.1.6 Fulguration of genital warts

Genital warts (HPV lesions, condylomata acuminata) were treated with fulguration in 48 young patients (42 male and 6 female, mean age±SD: 23.9 yrs ± 3.3). In the males the location of the warts varied: in most cases they involved the penile shaft skin and the preputial ridge, the inner layer of the prepuce, the frenular region and in 3 cases the glans penis. In the females the lesions were located at the vulvar region and in one case at the perineum. In cases of mucosal lesions topical anesthesia was achieved using a small quantity of EMLA cream (approximately 1-3 gr, depending on the extent of the lesions) and an occlusive dressing to keep the cream from being dislodged (Fig. 3). No dressing was used when the lesions were near hairy skin. In the cases of penile skin lesions and the perineal warts the dressing was left in place for 1 hour. The procedure was completed by fulguration of all visible lesions using the Birtcher Hyfercator at low power settings (approx. 5 Watts).

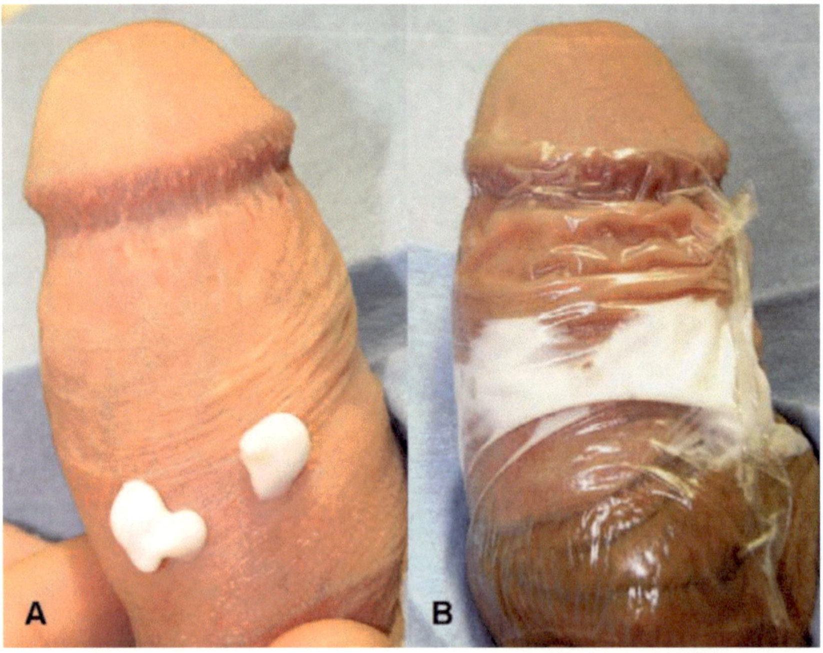

Fig. 3. Topical application of EMLA on penile HPV lesions (A). Placement of occlusive dressing (B).

2.1.7 Circumcision

A total of 68 male patients (mean age±SD: 47.8yrs ± 24.7) were subjected to circumcision due to phimosis. Topical anesthesia was initially achieved by spreading EMLA cream (approx. 2-5 gr) in the preputial sac with the aid of a 5 ml syringe. A plain cling film dressing was used for preventing the cream to spread out and the level of analgesia was evaluated first at 20 minutes and again at 30 minutes by pinching the prepuce with a toothed forceps. If the patient still reported pain or discomfort, further anesthesia was achieved initially by local infiltration with lignocaine (Xylocaine 2%, AstraZeneca Inc) at the ventral area (the frenular area). If this measure was inadequate, dorsal penile block with approximately 20 ml 1% Xylocaine was performed. After complete anesthesia was achieved, the foreskin was elevated, clamped with a straight forceps and cut until the glans was freed. Any redundant skin and inner prepuce were trimmed. Haemostasis was meticulously performed with diathermy and finally the edges of the skin and inner prepuce were sutured using absorbable sutures (3-0 polyglycolic acid, Safil QuickTM, B. Braun Melsungen AG). After completion of the procedure the traumatic surface was smeared with povidone iodine cream and a circular gauge dressing was applied leaving the urethra meatus free. The patient was advised on daily changes of the dressing and extra care of personal hygiene. No antibiotics or analgesics were prescribed.

3. Results

3.1 Effectiveness of topical anesthesia

A total of 321 patients were subjected to minor surgery of the external genitalia under topical anesthesia with EMLA cream. With the exception of circumcision patients, only one case in the short frenulum group and four cases in the genital warts group required further infiltration with local anesthetic. The overall satisfaction rate was excellent, as all patients were enthusiastic with the absence of needle pricks. All patients to whom anesthesia was sufficiently obtained with topical cream application stated that they would opt again for this type of local anesthesia for a similar procedure in the future. Detailed results for each type of procedure are presented below.

3.1.1 Separation of preputial adhesions

In all patients the use of EMLA cream obtained a sufficient level of anesthesia, allowing for completion of the procedure without need for further local anesthetic. However, anxiety of younger children did not allow for complete estimation of the level of local anesthesia, as we did not use formal monitoring of physiological parameters such as heart rate, respiratory rate etc. Nevertheless, we did not observe major symptoms of distress (excessive crying, protective movements) even in young boys (<20 months).

3.1.2 Short frenulum plasty

The level of local anesthesia obtained by EMLA cream in 20 minutes was sufficient in all cases except one. The latter was a patient with a notably thick frenulum who required further local anesthesia with lignocaine infiltration (~ 0.5 ml Xylocaine 2%) down the course of the procedure, while the deeper plate of the mucosa of the frenular bed was fulgurated for haemostasis. With the "pull and burn" method no sutures were generally used; in only three patients (2%) with a thick and wide frenulum, fine absorbable sutures (5-0 polyglycolic acid, Safil Quick™, B. Braun Melsungen AG) were used to approximate the lateral edges of the tear in order to achieve faster wound healing and better cosmetic result.

3.1.3 Meatotomy

The use of EMLA cream was in all cases sufficient to obtain a satisfactory level of local anesthesia until completion of the procedures. Even when sutures were used to anchor the urethral mucosa at the meatal lips, no pain was reported by the patients.

3.1.4 Fulguration of urethral warts

Topical EMLA application achieved a complete level of local anesthesia in all patients. Even when meatotomy was performed in order to gain access to warts rooted deeply in the fossa navicularis, no further anesthesia was necessary.

3.1.5 Urethral prolapse correction

The intraurethral application of EMLA cream was in all cases sufficient to obtain a satisfactory level of local anesthesia until completion of the procedures. Only one woman reported minor discomfort while the urethral mucosa was sutured to the meatus; however this was well tolerated and no further infiltrative anesthesia was required.

3.1.6 Fulguration of genital warts

Generally, warts on mucosal surface (penile, vulvar) were removed under topical cream anesthesia. In 4 out of 9 cases (45%) of warts located on penile and perianal skin further infiltration with 2% lignocaine was required. However in three of these cases which were men with condylomata located at the penile shaft skin near the pubis, the occlusive dressing had been dislocated during the waiting time of 1 hour, as pubic hair did not allow for air-tight adhesion of the Tegaderm® dressing. In the rest of 44 patients (91.67%) no further local anesthetic was required and fulguration was completed uneventfully.

3.1.7 Circumcision

In only 14/68 cases (20.5%) with phimosis the use of topical cream alone was sufficient for anesthesia until completion of the procedure. Although not properly classified, our impression is that these patients featured a limited area of foreskin, which was thin and elastic. In the rest of the 54 patients (79.5%) further local infiltration with 2% lignocaine was required in 21 cases (38.9%) and dorsal penile nerve block with 1% lignocaine was required in 33 cases (61.1%). The use of EMLA cream in most of these cases would alleviate to some extent the painful stimuli (e.g. clamping with forceps); however this was not adequate for completion of the procedure and the patients required further analgesia.

3.2 Complications and side effects

A sensation of "mint freshness" was reported by most patients when the cream was applied on mucosal surface. Local erythema was present in almost all cases with mucosal application; however this did not affect the course of the procedures. No significant skin reaction or allergic reaction occurred in any patient. No systematic reactions, cyanosis or methemoglobinaemia were recorded, even in the group of young boys undergoing separation of preputial adhesions.

4. Discussion

The development of topical anesthetics in the latter half of the 19th century was a revolution in local anesthesia. Today pain can be alleviated for a wide variety of minor procedures on intact or even lacerated skin and mucosa. This evolution in topical cream anesthetics has offered surgeons, plastic surgeons and even family medicine physicians a useful tool in treating several conditions safely at an office setting. In the genitourinary surgery setting, these procedures include (but are not limited to): circumcision, preputial plasty and frenulum plasty, meatotomy and meatal dilatation, removal of genital warts by curettage, fulguration, laser surgery or cryotherapy, biopsies of genital skin and mucosa, separation of preputial adhesions in boys and hymenal or labial adhesions in girls. In the past, most types of these procedures would require infiltration with a local anesthetic such as lignocaine and at least some form of sedation. The use of topical acting anesthetics is patient-friendly as they eliminate needle fear and anxiety and injection pain at the beginning of the procedure. Moreover the minor skin reactions observed (local erythema or minor oedema) are an advantage over infiltrative anesthetics which often produce bleeding, heamatomas or oedema that may distort the surgical site, a fact that may be important in delicate procedures with a desired good aesthetic result. One should also bear in mind the always present risk of accidental systemic intravascular injection of injectables, especially in procedures where higher doses of local anesthetic are needed. In this series we have used EMLA cream, a eutectic mixture of local anesthetics, 2.5% lidocaine and 2.5% prilocaine, to provide local anesthesia for a variety of surgical procedures at the external genitalia of children, men and women at an office setting.

4.1 Topical anesthetics

EMLA has not been the first topical anesthetic to be used in the office setting. After the initial enthusiasm for cocaine as a topical anesthetic, a series of mixtures have been developed in an effort to produce an effective and safe topical compound. Tetracaine, adrenaline and cocaine (TAC), a compound of 0.5% tetracaine, 0.05% epinephrine and 11.8% cocaine was the first mixture of topical anesthetics to be effective for skin lacerations (Kundu, 2002). A small amount of this solution (2-5 ml) is applied directly to the wound with a cotton tip and maintained under pressure for 20-40 minutes. However concerns about toxicity, expence and legal issues regarding cocaine have led the medical community to abandon its use (Kundu, 2002).

An alternative to TAC (with cocaine substituted by lignocaine) was LET, a compound of 0.5% tetracaine, 0.1% epinephrine and 4% lignocaine (Xylocaine). This mixture has to be formulated as a liquid or gel. No severe side-effects have been reported but care should be taken when used in end-arterioral areas of the body due to the effect of epinephrine. Moreover, mucosal application should be avoided. Other newer compounds developed include LMX-4 and LMX-5 (which contain liposomal lignocaine 4% or 5% respectively) and

BLT (a triple anesthetic gel consisting of 20% benzocaine, 6% lignocaine and 4% tetracaine). Iontophoresis is another method that can transfer medications into the skin through the use of constant, low-voltage direct current. In this setting, sponges soaked in lignocaine are applied on intact skin and the current is applied, producing a good anesthetic effect that lasts for 42 to 110 minutes (Kaweski, 2008). However there are limits to this method too. Skin burns may occur if the current is set too high, special equipment and training are necessary and the area to be anaesthetized can only be small and flat. Moreover, it has not been used on mucosal surfaces.

EMLA cream is an oil-in-water emulsion of 2.5% lignocaine and 2.5% prilocaine. The eutectic mixture contains a thickener, an emulsifier and distilled water adjusted to a pH level of 9.4 (Kundu, 2002). This formulation enhances absorption through intact skin. For our group of patients EMLA seemed the best choice, due to its commercial availability, low cost and easiness in application. Moreover EMLA has been successfully used on genital mucosa, despite initial concerns of prilocaine absorption. It should be noted however that other topical anesthetics may give comparable results as they all share common action mechanisms.

4.2 Mechanism of action

For a topical anesthetic to act it must firstly penetrate the outer barriers of the body, eg the epidermis or the mucosal surface in order to reach the deeper dermal layers of the skin, concentrate in the vicinity of pain receptors and free nerve endings and eventually penetrate the individual axons in the nerve. Local anesthetics generally feature a lipid-soluble hydrophobic aromatic group (aromatic ring), an intermediate ester and a charged, hydrophilic group (terminal amine). Greater lipid solubility enhances diffusion through nerve sheaths as well as neural membranes of individual axons. Both lignocaine and prilocaine contained in EMLA cream are amide type anesthetics, which accounts for their stability, heat resistance and low allergenic potential (Edgcombe, n.d.). These local anesthetics act through interruption of the neural conduction through inhibition of the influx of sodium ions (Becker, 2006).

Normal neural conduction is based on the ability of neural tissue to become excitable in an electrical sense and further conduct the initial impulse. This is mediated through fluctuations of the ionic gradients that normally exist across the axonal membrane. At the resting phase, a potential of about 70mV (resting potential) is generated by the constant activity of a sodium-potassium pump which continuously pumps out sodium to the outside of the membrane while potassium is being pumped in. The result is marked concentration difference (concentration gradient) for these two cations across the axonal membrane (Neilson, n.d.). Depolarisation of the membrane is triggered by sudden opening of sodium channels, resulting in a massive influx of Na. This in turn produces a rise in membrane potential to around 40mV.Repolarisation occurs through closure of sodium channels in the presence of continuous efflux of potassium. As the intracellular potential falls back to its resting levels, the potassium channels close in turn. This depolarization wave is propagated and the impulses are transmitted across the axon.

Local anesthetics disrupt ion channel function within the neuronal membrane. This is occurring by specific binding of the anesthetic molecule to the sodium channels. The channels are held in an inactive state, preventing further depolarization of the membrane. The action of the molecule in its ionized form is exerted from *within* the cell i.e. the anesthetic has to cross the neuronal membrane in order to block the sodium channels. The effect of the anesthetic is not limited to pain reduction; the loss of nerve function also includes loss of temperature, touch, proprioception and eventually muscle tone (Edgcombe, n.d)

The time for onset of local anesthesia is regulated by the amount of unionized drug present at physiological pH (7.4). As all local anesthetics are weak bases, they exist in both ionized and unionized form. The dissociation constant (pKa) of a local anesthetic determines the amount of an administered dose that exists in an ionized form at any given pH. The lower the pKa, the greater the proportion in the tertiary, diffusible state, a fact that in turn hastens onset of action. Lignocaine for example has a pKa of 7.9 while bupivacaine has a pKa of 8.1, hence lignocaine is approximately 25% (versus 15% for bupivacaine) unionized at pH 7.4, a fact that explains lignocaine's more rapid onset of action. Prilocaine has also a pKa of 7.9, hence the formulation of EMLA has two equally fast acting local anesthetics.

4.3 Application

The method of application of EMLA cream is straightforward and easy. According to the product datasheet, a thick layer of cream is applied on intact skin and covered with an occlusive dressing, either a self-adhesive e.g. Tegaderm® or plain cling film. The purpose is to create an air-tight environment that facilitates absorption of the cream ingredients. After minimum one hour (1 hr) the dressing is removed and any excess cream has to be cleaned thoroughly prior to the procedure. For skin applications the suggested dose is $1.5gr/cm^2$ and maximum application time is 5 hours. For mucosal applications, the suggested dose is even higher, approximately 2gr per lesion, with a maximum of 10 gr. The suggested waiting time is 5-10 minutes. An occlusive dressing is not necessary (EMLA product monograph).

In our cases with skin lesions such as penile skin warts and circumcision we used the recommended dose for 1 hour in all cases, along with an occlusive dressing. Other investigators have used even higher doses on skin applications (Laffon, 1998; Buckley & Benfield, 1993). When treating lesions on mucosal surfaces (penile or vulvar) we used the smallest quantity necessary and not the recommended dose. An occlusive dressing was used on mucosal surfaces as well (either Tegaderm® or plain cling film) although not suggested. The reason for the dressing was not to create an air-tight barrier but rather to prevent the cream from being dislodged while the patient relaxed in the waiting room. In cases of vulvar lesions where no dressing was applicable the patients had to wait in the office surgery, usually in a modified lithotomy position. The time allowed for the cream to act on mucosal surfaces was generally 20 minutes. The recommended time is 5-10 minutes; however from our previous experience this amount of time is not always sufficient for achieving a satisfactory level of local anesthesia, especially for procedures such as frenulum plasty or large condylomata in which deeper levels of the preputial mucosa had to be fulgurated. Other studies have suggested that the quality of analgesia actually *decreases* with application times longer than 10 to 15 minutes (Zilbert, 2002). This decreased efficacy associated with longer periods of application time is attributed to lidocaine-induced vasodilatation and subsequent increased systemic absorption (Kundu, 2002). However this negative time effect has not been verified in our series.

When the EMLA cream was delivered into the urethral meatus (e.g. in urethral warts, meatotomy and urethral prolapse) we used a small syringe to administer the desired dose. This was much easier than using small probes or cannulation catheters we had used in the past. One has to be careful to remove all air bubbles from the syringe before squeezing the cream. A time lap of 20 minutes was in all cases sufficient for achieving an adequate level of anesthesia.

The use of EMLA in the pediatric population warrants special precautions. The suggested dose for infants 3 up to 12 months is up to 2 gr, for approximately 1 hour. For children 1-6 years and >10kg the dose increases up to 10 gr. However these refer to skin applications (EMLA product monograph). No standardized doses for mucosal applications are available. However several studies have used EMLA cream for topical anesthesia in the preputial sac, for procedures such as circumcision, meatotomy and release of preputial adhesions (Smith, 2004; Ben-Meir, 2011; Butler-O'Hara, 1998). The doses used varied from 0.5 to 2gr and the application time extended from 30 mins to 1 hour. In our cases of preputial adhesions we used a cotton tip to deliver the cream inside the preputial sac and tried to use the minimum amount possible (0.5-1gr). In most cases the anesthetic effect was already demonstrable at 20 mins.

4.4 Efficacy

In our series the EMLA cream provided excellent topical anesthesia when mucosal surfaces were treated. In the majority of adult cases where mucosal lesions were involved, local anesthesia was thorough and allowed for completion of the procedure without the need for further infiltrative anesthetic. Only one patient with an extra thick frenulum required further lignocaine injection during the procedure. Our results verify the excellent anesthetic effect of EMLA on the genital mucosa. Similar results have been demonstrated with EMLA use in procedures such as frenuloplasty or meatotomy (Laffon, 1998; Buckley & Benfield, 1993; Ben-Meir, 2011). However, the above mentioned results are not directly comparable, as the above mentioned investigators also used other forms of analgesia or sedation (e.g. nitrous oxide).

When EMLA was applied on skin lesions, the results were not so impressive. In 4 cases with genital warts the degree of anesthesia was insufficient and further local anesthetic (2% Xylocaine) had to be injected on site. Of course a "relieving" explanation in three of these cases would be the dislodgment of the cream from the penile skin; however even in these cases enough cream was left in place for a positive result to occur. Failures were most prominent in the group of phimosis patients undergoing circumcision. In only 20.5% of these patients topical anesthesia was adequate for completion of the procedure. In the majority of the circumcision cases (79.5%) additional local infiltration with 2% Xylocaine or dorsal penile nerve block with 1% Xylocaine was necessary. Similar results have been reported by other authors in both adult and pediatric populations undergoing circumcision (Laffon, 1998; Butler-O'Hara, 1998) .It appears that the complex innervation of the penile skin and prepuce does not allow for the use of a topical cream as a sole anesthetic agent. In the case of a proper circumcision, three parts of the penis have to be anesthetized: the penile shaft skin, the inner layer of the prepuce and especially the ridged band and the mostly sensitive frenular area. This may explain why application of EMLA on the inner part of the preputial sac is firstly incomplete (due to phimosis) and secondly inadequate to provide anesthesia to the penile shaft skin. Even combined application (i.e. administration to both the preputial sac and the shaft skin with occlusive dressing) has not been proved adequate (personal unpublished data). It is of interest that only in cases with a thin, soft prepuce (although this can not be properly measured) the EMLA cream provided sufficient analgesia. It is possible that penetration of the anesthetics was easier through a thinner mucosal epithelium and lamina propria of the prepuce. Nevertheless it should be noted that although EMLA was insufficient for initiation or completion of the procedure it did however partly alleviate the pain from further local infiltration. This finding suggests that EMLA may be used as an agent for pain reduction associated with local infiltration or dorsal penile nerve block during circumcision.

In our pediatric population the effect of EMLA on pain reduction during release of preputial adhesions is deemed effective. Although we did not use proper tools such as Visual Analog Scale (VAS), the Wong-Baker Faces scale or Neonatal Infant Pain Scale (NIPS), behavioral responses (facial activity, time spent crying, protective movement) were recorded during the procedures. However it is rather difficult to correctly estimate the effect of EMLA in this setting as the anxiety of certain young patients (or the anxiety of the parents!) may obscure the effect of the local anesthetic. In our series every care was taken to reassure the patients that no pain would be present and that they just had to stay relaxed and tranquil. The effect of the parents' presence was equivocal, depending on the character of the child. Keeping these variables in mind, we considered the topical anesthetic effective when no major signs of distress (excessive crying, protective movements, quick breathing) were present during the procedure and the patient himself tolerated the procedure until completion.

4.5 Adverse effects

No major adverse effects were present in any case in this series. In the adult population only topical signs of a transient erythema were present in almost all cases of mucosal application. This biphasic skin reaction of blanching and erythema is thought to occur due to initial peripheral vasoconstriction followed by vasodilatation (Kaweski, 2008). In any case this is a negligible side effect that does not affect the surgical site. Most of our patients reported that the erythema disappeared within 1-2 hours. A mild sensation of burning and itching has also been reported in several studies (Zilbert, 2002). In our series most patients only reported a "freshmint" sensation at the site of application. Rarely contact dermatitis may develop secondary to prilocaine (Kaweski, 2008). Another rare but potentially lethal complication of local anesthetics is methemoglobinemia.

Methemoglobin (metHb) is produced when within the hemoglobin molecule ferrous iron is oxidized to ferric iron. This effect impairs oxygen transport to tissues (Boran, 2008). MetHb is normally maintained at concentrations below 2% of total hemoglobin, due to the activity of NADH dehydrogenase which reduces metHb to hemoglobin. Neonates are most prone to develop methemoglobinemia because the cytochrome b5 reductase level in infants is only 50% of adult values and methemoglobin can accumulate. Several drugs may induce methemoglobinemia, such as sulfonamides, nitrofurantoin, nitrates, phenytoin, phenacetin, phenobarbital and others. As far as EMLA is concerned, a metabolite of prilocaine called o-toluidine is known to induce methemoglobinemia (EMLA product monograph).

The initial presentation of an infant with mild methemoglobinemia is characterized by tissue cyanosis, a bluish-grey discoloration of the skin, especially around lips and nail beds, palor or marbleization. It is characteristic that this cyanotic picture is not reversed by administration of 100% oxygen. Severe methemoglobinemia (concentrations above 25%) presents with seizures, cardiovascular collapse and coma. Severe methemoglobinemia represents an emergency; first-line antidote is methylene blue, a thiazide dye that accelerates the enzymatic reduction of metHb by NADHP reductase and also acts as scavenger for free radicals (Boran, 2008). However when methylene blue is not readily available, intravenous high doses of ascorbic acid may be used as an alternative.

4.6 Safety concerns

Topical anesthetic creams are generally safe and effective when used appropriately. In the past deaths have occurred when anesthetic creams compounded in formulas with non-standard doses were used by inexperienced personnel or even self-applied by patients (Kaweski, 2008). EMLA cream is a standard dose compound, with many years of clinical use. The recommended doses should be respected and the application time not exceeded significantly. In our series we used the smallest amount possible, especially on mucosal application. The recorded effectiveness of EMLA cream in these cases, even with doses smaller than suggested, demonstrates that the anesthetic effect is not necessarily associated with a "thick layer" of cream, as originally described in the product's datasheet (EMLA product monograph). Every effort should be made to limit the skin or mucosal area covered to the smaller extent necessary. EMLA cream is not intended for use on large areas. Special precautions should be used in specific cases. A history of congenital or idiopathic methemoglobinemia is an absolute contraindication; patients with glucose-6-phosphate dehydrogenase (G-6-P-D) deficiency and those who require treatment with methemoglobin - inducing drugs are more susceptible to acquired methemoglobinemia.

The use of EMLA in the pediatric population should follow the general rules on dosage and application time with a special focus on the increased vulnerability of infants to methemoglobinemia. Topical use of EMLA should be avoided in infants less than 3 months and other sedation or anesthetic alternatives should be preferred for this age group. Moreover, when EMLA cream is used for topical anesthesia, children should be closely monitored during and after the procedure for early signs of complications such as methemoglobinemia. In our series no such an event occurred. Nevertheless the children with preputial adhesions were kept and monitored in the waiting room for at least one hour after completion of the procedure and the parents and caretakers were thoroughly advised on which signs they should become alert during the following hours.

5. Conclusions

The use of topical anesthetic creams has gained popularity in the recent years over injectable local anesthetics due to the advantage of needle pain and anxiety elimination. In our series of patients the application of EMLA cream as a topical anesthetic proved to be a useful, efficient and safe tool for minor surgical procedures of the external genitalia in children, men and women at the office setting. Side effects can be kept to a minimum when the amount used is limited (especially at mucosal application) and the time allowed for action is carefully tailored to the site of application, patient's age and type of procedure.

6. References

Becker D, Reed K. Essentials of local anesthetic Pharmacology. Anesth Prog Vol. 53, (2006), pp. 98-108.

Ben-Meir D, Livne PM, Feigin E, Djerassi R. & Efrat R. Meatotomy using local anesthesia and sedation or general anesthesia with or without penile block in children: a prospective randomized study. *J Urol* Vol 185, No.2, (Feb 2010), pp. 654-657.

Boran P., Tokuc G., & Yegin Z. methemoglobinemia due to application of prilocaine during circumcision and the effect of ascorbic acid. Journal of pediatric *Urology*. Vol.1 No4 (2008), pp.475-476.

Buckley M., Benfield P. Eutectic Lidocaine/Prilocaine cream: A review of the topical anaesthetic/analgesic efficacy of a Eutectic Mixture of Local Anaesthetics (EMLA). *Drugs*, Vol.46, No.1 (July 1993), pp.126-151.

Butler-O'Hara M, LeMoine C. & Guillet R. Analgesia for neonatal circumcision: arandomized controlled trial of EMLA cream versus dorsal penile nerve block. *Pediatrics*, Vol. 101, No 4, (1998), e5.

Cold CJ, Taylor JR. The prepuce. *British Journal of Urology*, Vol 83, Suppl. No 1, (1999), pp. 34-44.

Edgcombe H. Local anaesthetic pharmacology. Available from: http://www.frca.co.uk/printfriendly.aspx?articleid=100505

EMLA product monograph. Date of revision: May 5, 2010. Available from: http://www.astrazeneca.ca.

Gordetsky J, Bendana E, OBrien J, & Rabinowitz R. (Almost) painless surgery: a historical review of the evolution of intraurethral anesthesia in Urology. *Urology*, Vol.77, No 1, (2011), pp.12-16.

Gyftopoulos K. Male dyspareunia due to short frenulum: the suture-free, "pull and burn" method. *Journal of Sexual Medicine* Vol.6, No9 (September 2009), pp. 2611-2614.

Kaweski S. Topical Anesthetic creams. *Plastic & Reconstructive Surgery Journal*. Vol.121, No.6, (June 2008), pp. 2161-6165.

Kundu S, Achar S. Principles of office anesthesia: PartII. Topical anesthesia. *American Family Physician*. Vol.66, No1, (July 2002), pp. 99-102.

Laffon M, Gouchet A, Quenum M, Haillot O, Mercier C. & Huguet M. Eutectic mixture of local anesthetics in adult urology patients: an observational trial. *Regional Anesthesia Pain Med*icine. Vol. 23, No.5, (Sep-Oct 1998), pp. 502-5.

Neilson A. Mechanism of action of local anaesthetics. Available from: http://www.csaol.cn/img/hypertextbook/a/c53.htm

Smith DP, Gjellum M. The efficacy od LMX versus EMLA for pain relief in boys undergoing office meatotomy. *J Urol* Vol 172, No 4, (Oct 2004), pp. 1760-1761.

Zilbert A. Topical anesthesia for minor gynaecological procedures: A review. *Obstetrical and Gynaecological Survey*. Vol57, No.3, (2002), pp. 171-178.